Current Research in Endometriosis

Current Research in Endometriosis

Edited by **Chris Flagstad**

New Jersey

Published by Foster Academics,
61 Van Reypen Street,
Jersey City, NJ 07306, USA
www.fosteracademics.com

Current Research in Endometriosis
Edited by Chris Flagstad

International Standard Book Number: 978-1-63242-101-2 (Hardback)

Printed in the United States of America.

Contents

Preface

This comprehensive book consists of research-focused information in respect of endometriosis. It offers to provide an understanding of the developing trends in progress, diagnosis and management of endometriosis. This book provides an overview of endometriosis and discusses latest research reports on infertility, endometrial receptivity, ovarian cancer and altered gene expression associated with endometriosis; various predictive markers and imaging modalities including MRI and ultrasound for efficient diagnosis as well as current non-hormonal and hormonal treatment strategies. This book will prove to be a valuable and rich resource for clinicians, scientists and students who are interested in gaining an improved understanding of endometriosis and also interested in recent research trends related to the disease.

This book unites the global concepts and researches in an organized manner for a comprehensive understanding of the subject. It is a ripe text for all researchers, students, scientists or anyone else who is interested in acquiring a better knowledge of this dynamic field.

I extend my sincere thanks to the contributors for such eloquent research chapters. Finally, I thank my family for being a source of support and help.

Editor

Section 1

Recent Research Trends

Primary Afferent Nociceptors and Visceral Pain

Victor Chaban

Charles R. Drew University of Medicine and Science and
University of California, Los Angeles,
USA

1. Introduction

Patients with chronic pelvic pain frequently have pain from several pelvic organs. The most common diagnoses include endometriosis, interstitial cystitis, irritable bowel disease, pelvic floor tension myalgia, vulvar vestibulitis, and vulvodynia. Frequently, pain does not correlate with pathologic findings at the time of laparoscopy in the case of endometriosis, while vulvodynia, irritable bowel syndrome and pelvic floor tension myalgia and neuropathy may have no clearly demonstrable pathologic tissue changes. Most diagnoses associated with chronic pelvic pain have a high rate of recurrence and all are considered to be chronic conditions with a relapsing course. Endometriosis is a complex, poorly understood chronic illness of women in their reproductive age and pain is the major concern of women with this disease. Despite a successful reduction of pain using during the novel treatments pain returns in up to 75% of treated women. Pain is strongly associated with this disease and the lack of awareness to its pathology is further illustrated by the fact that the average time duration between the onset of pain and the diagnosis of endometriosis is 3 to 11 years despite the fact that 25-30% of women with chronic pelvic pain suffer from this disease. In women with endometriosis (mainly of reproductive age) alterations in the limbic and sympathetic nervous system and hypothalamic-pituitary-adrenal axis mediate a cycle of hypervigilance for pain sensations from pelvic organs, which can lead to descending induction of pathologic changes in pelvic organs. Chronic pelvic pain patients frequently have multiple diagnoses. Vicero-somatic and viscero-viseral hyperalgesia and allodynia result in the spread of a perception of pain from an initial site to adjacent areas. Chronic pelvic pain patients may initially have only one pain source in the pelvis, such as the uterus in dysmenorrhea or endometriosis implants, but a multitude of mechanisms involving the peripheral and central nervous system can lead to the development of painful sensations from other adjacent organs. Often the etiology of visceral pain is not clear, as there are many symptoms of the reproductive system, gastrointestinal and urinary tracts, musculoskeletal, neurological and psychological systems that often co-occur in the same patient. The variation of pain symptoms and pain perception and behavioral responses to pain in these patients is poorly understood. The treating clinician is often tempted to take a unidimensional approach and focus on one organ system and ignore the psychological and behavioral manifestations of the chronic pain.

The incidence of persistent, episodic, or chronic visceral pain are more prevalent in females thus defining the site(s) and mechanisms through which female steroid hormones modulate visceral nociception is an important step in understanding the gender differences in pain perception and in designing appropriate therapies for females. One such mechanism may be the convergence of nociceptive stimuli and estrogen input on the primary afferent neurons which innervate viscera. Based on our results, it is likely that estrogen receptors (ERs) expressed in primary afferent neurons modulate nociceptive signaling. Our recent data suggest that estrogen acting on primary afferent nociceptors modulates the response to pro- and anti-nociceptive signals associated with the clinical presentation of functional disorders such as endometriosis.

1.2 The nociception of endometriosis

Endometrial tissues outside the uterus can cause severe pain and this pain can be diminished with therapies that suppress estrogen production (Berkley *et al.* 2005). The mechanism of endometriosis-induced nociceptive signaling is poorly understood and in some cases pain can be exacerbated by co-morbidity with other chronic pelvic pain syndromes such as irritable bowel syndrome, painful bladder syndrome, vulvodynia and fibromyalgia. It has also been shown that ectopic implants develop sensory nerve supply both in women and in animal models of endometriosis. Sensory input arriving from the visceral organ to the spinal cord divergences at the level of primary sensory neurons which further transmit considerable information from periphery to the central nervous system. Visceral pain may be manifestation from a single organ such as uterus or may arise from algogenic conditions affecting more than one organ (Malykhina 2007). This type of pain is important not only because it is difficult to diagnose its clinical conditions but also for its therapeutic implications. It is quite possible to modulate pain from one viscus to another. Recent study by Giamberardino and others showed that the treatment of the endometriotic lesions results in the improvement of spontaneous and referred urinary symptoms (Giamberardino *et al.* 2010).

Cross-sensitization in the pelvis implies the transmission of noxious stimuli from one organ to another through an adjacent normal structure resulting in functional (rarely organic) changes. Pelvic organ cross-sensitization is considered as one of the factors contributing to chronic pelvic pain (Pezzone *et al.* 2005). Chronic pelvic pain (CPP) syndrome affects up to 25% of reproductive age women and results in dysmenorrhea, menstrual irregularities, back pain and reduced fecundity. One of the most common causes of CPP is endometriosis. Chronic pain adversely affects mood, social and professional life and general well being. Thus, assessing the impact of the pain on various domains of a patient's existence has become an important focus in the clinical management. Most women with complaints of pelvic pain will undergo laparoscopy to both diagnose and treat these diseases, but laparoscopy is often is unsuccessful due to lack of intraperitoneal pathology or altered pain processing. Pain out of proportion to identifiable pathology is the most immediate and dramatic consequence of disorders associated with CPP and is responsible for a highly negative impact on quality of life and substantial workforce loss. Results of a national survey determined that 15% of women in the United States have experienced CPP and only 10% of these consulted a gynecologist and 75% did not consult a health care provider of any type. Due to the alarming situation and unmet need, the USA and other countries have launched a call for more focused research on improving the diagnosis and treatment of CPP syndrome.

There is often no clear relationship between the severity of the chronic pelvic pain and pathology in the pelvic viscera, including reproductive tract (ovaries and uterus). It is still poorly understood how endometriosis is associated with pain symptoms in different organs and how this nociceptive signaling is ameliorated by a hypoestrogenic state. One of the possible explanation can be that endometrial implants' sensory nerve supply and its potentially estradiol-modulated influence on the nociception.

Several researchers have investigated the presence of nerve fibers in endometriotic lesions in both human and animal study. Using different types of specific immunohistochemical neuronal markers such as substance P (SP) and calcitonin gene related peptide (CGRP) sensory nerve fibers markers) in human peritoneal endometriotic lesions from women with visually and biopsy proven endometriosis, investigators have demonstrated multiple, small unmyelinated nerve fibers are present in peritoneal endometriotic lesions, and these peritoneal endometriotic lesions contain both Aδ and C nerve fibers. Accumulating evidence has shown these nerve fibers may play a critical role in pain production in patients with endometriosis, and a close histological relationship has been identified between these nerve fibers and endometriosis associated pain. Tulandi *et al.* (2001) reported that the distance between endometriotic glands and nerve fibers in endometriotic lesions from women with pain was closer than in women with no pain. The density of nerve fibers in peritoneal endometriotic lesions was much greater than in normal peritoneum in women with no endometriosis. The nerve fiber density in endometriotic lesions can be markedly reduced by hormonal drugs such as gonadotropin releasing hormone (GnRH) analogues and combined oral contraceptives, which have been used efficaciously to treat endometriosis-associated pain, indicating that modulation of these nerve fibers might alter pelvic nociception. The fact that peritoneal endometriotic lesions are innervated by sensory Aδ, sensory C nerve fibers raises the intriguing questions, what kind of role do these nerve fibers play in the mechanisms by which endometriotic lesions produce pain and hyperalgesia, and how do they modulate pain perception in these condition?

The demonstration of Aδ and C sensory fiber innervations to peritoneal endometriotic lesions, suggesting these innervations contributes to both visceral hyperalgesia and pelvic pain that occur in patients with endometriosis brings up the interesting questions, how do these sensory fibers transmit and modulate visceral nociception in endometriosis? Immunohistochemical staining of these nerve fibers in endometriosis showed co-localization of SP, CGRP, implicating SP and CGRP might be involved in modulation of visceral nociception. Endometriosis is an inflammatory disease, which is known to contain pro-inflammatory cytokines, prostaglandins, and other neuroactive agents that could readily activate the CGRP- and SP-positive C-fiber nociceptive afferents found in the endometriotic lesions.

When these sensory nerve fibers are stimulated by inflammatory substances, neurotransmitters such as SP, CGRP can be secreted from sensory nerve endings. SP and CGRP can contribute to the inflammatory response by causing vasodilation, plasma extravasation and cellular infiltration by interacting with endothelial cells, arterioles, mast cells, neutrophils and immune cells. SP can also act on mast cells in the vicinity of sensory nerve endings to evoke de-granulation and the release of TNF-α, histamine, prostaglandin D2 (PGD2) and leukotriene, providing a positive feedback. CGRP has a wide range of biological activities, including sensory transmission, regulation of glandular secretion, and inhibiting SP degradation by a specific endopeptidase to enhance SP release, thereby amplifying the effects.

Dorsal root ganglion (DRG) neurons can be activated or modulated by the activation of chemosensitive receptors on peripheral terminals and ATP has been implicated in sensory transduction of noxious stimuli by activating purinergic P2X receptors (Dunn *et al.* 2001). Once released into the intercellular areas, the action of ATP is mediated by primarily P2X3 receptors which are expressed on primary afferent fibers and cell bodies within DRG (Burnstock 2001). The capsaicin-sensitive primary afferent neurons of small- and medium-diameter neurons mediate nociceptive-like behaviors suggesting that TRPV1 expressing neurons are nociceptors. Activation of purinergic (P2X3) and transient potential receptors family vcanilloid-1 (TRPV1) receptors results in the depolarization and opening of voltage-gated Ca^{2+}channels (VGCC) (Koshimizu *et al.* 2000). A sensation of pain is produced by depolarization of the peripheral nerve terminals.

1.3 Estrogen receptors and nociceptive signaling in primary afferent neurons

Defining the site(s) and mechanisms through which sex estrogen modulates visceral nociception is an important step in understanding the mechanisms in pain perception associated with endometriosis and in designing appropriate therapies. One such mechanism may be the convergence of nociceptive stimuli and estrogen input on the primary afferent neurons which innervate viscera (i.e. uterus). Estrogen may modulate female sensitivity to clinical and experimentally induced pain. Based on our preliminary results, it is likely that estrogen receptors (ERs) expressed in primary afferent neurons modulate chemical signaling associated with nociception. Nociception is a balance of pro- and anti-nociceptive inputs that is subject to regulation depending on the normal state of the organism. Sensitization of primary afferent neurons to stimulation may play a role in the enhanced perception of visceral sensation and pain. Chest pain from coronary heart disease, endometriosis, acute and recurrent/chronic pelvic pain in women or abdominal are all visceral pain sensations that may result in part from sensitization (Berkley *et al.* 2001; Mayer *et al.* 2001). Mechanisms of peripheral sensitization may involve increased transduction that is secondary to repeated stimulation or an increase in the excitability of the afferent nerves by molecules that decrease the excitation threshold (Zimmermann 2001)

The cell bodies of primary visceral spinal afferent neurons are located in DRG. Direct activation of chemosensitive receptors and ion channels on their peripheral terminals and modulation of neuronal excitability activates extrinsic primary afferent nerves. Nociceptors belong predominantly to small and medium size DRG neurons whose peripheral processes detect potentially damaging physical and chemical stimuli. The terminals of primary visceral afferent neurons are described as having no organs end or morphological specialization, but respond to different chemical stimuli. Visceral nociceptive C-fibers activated by ATP released by noxious stimuli from cells in target organs, have been implicated as mediators of noxious stimulus intensities (Burnstock 2000). Alteration in signal transduction of primary afferent neurons can result in enhanced perception of the visceral sensation that is common in patients with different disorders resulting in elevated pain perception. Acute and recurrent/chronic pelvic pain in women and abdominal pain from IBS are illustrative examples of visceral pain that undergo sensitization (Giamberardino *et al.* 2010).

Peripheral sensitization can develop in response to sustain stimulation, inflammation, and nerve injury. Visceral pain is different from cutaneous pain based on clinical, neurophysiological and pharmacological characteristics (Chang and Heitkemper 2002). The pathophysiology of visceral hyperalgesia is less well-known than its cutaneous counterpart, and our understanding of visceral hyperalgesia is colored by comparison to cutaneous hyperalgesia, which is believed to arise as a consequence of the sensitization of peripheral nociceptors due to long-lasting changes in the excitability of spinal neurons. Endometriosis is currently defined as a chronic functional syndrome characterized by recurring symptoms of abdominal discomfort or pain. In the context of visceral pain, the TRPV1 receptor is a sensory neuron-specific cation channel which plays an important role in transporting thermal and inflammatory pain signals. Evidence for TRPV1's role is that mice lacking TRP1 receptor gene have deficits in thermal- or inflammatory-induced hyperalgesia (Davis *et al.* 2000). Activation of both TRPV1 and P2X receptors induce mobilization of $[Ca^{2+}]_i$ in cultured DRG neurons (Gschossmann *et al.* 2000).

Sex hormones and 17β-estradiol (E2) in particular may directly influence the functions of primary afferent neurons since both ERs are present on small-diameter DRG neurons (Papka and Storey-Workley 2002). Despite the broad spectrum of E2 effects in the nervous system, the mechanisms of hormonal pain modulation remain unclear. There are two subforms: estrogen receptor-α (ERα) and estrogen receptor-β (ERβ) which were traditionally thought of as ligand-activated transcription factors. However, recent work has demonstrated multiplicity of E_2 actions (membrane, cytoplasmic and nuclear) (Nadal *et al.* 2001). ER distributed through CNS and PNS including regions that mediate nociception. For example, ERs are expressed in dorsal horn neurons of the spinal cord and DRG neurons. DRG neurons express both ERα and ERβ *in vivo* (Papka and Storey-Workley 2002) and *in vitro* (Chaban 2010). These findings suggest that E2 may modulate sensory input at the primary afferent level. E2 can alter gene transcription, resulting in pro-nociceptive (reducing β-endorphin expression) or anti-nociceptive (increasing enkephalin expression) changes of endogenous opioid peptides , opioid receptors (Micevych and Sinchak 2001) and, by increasing levels of CCK, an anti-nociceptive and anti-opioid molecule (Micevych *et al.* 2002).

E2 can modulate cellular activity by altering ion channel opening and second messenger signaling by stimulating G-proteins (Chaban *et al.* 2003) , the signal transduction pathways traditionally associated with membrane receptor activation. Many of these effects have been ascribed to membrane-associated receptors. The results from other laboratories (Lee *et al.* 2002) and our data (Chaban *et al.* 2003) indicate that E2 is acting to modulate L-type VGCC. The cloned TRPV1 receptor is a nonselective cation channel with a high permeability for Ca^{2+}. TRPV1's are distributed in peripheral sensory nerve endings and are involved in the transduction of different stimuli in sensory neurons. TRPV1 functions as molecular integrator of painful chemical and physical stimuli (noxious heat (>43° C) and low pH). Various inflammatory mediators such as prostaglandin E_2 (PGE2) and bradykinin potentiate TRPV1. The potentiation of TRPV1 activity can be quantified by measuring the differences of capsaicin-induced Ca^{2+} concentration changes before and after receptor activation (Petruska *et al.* 2000). Significantly, a subset of DRG neurons respond to both capsaicin and ATP indicating that there may be cross-activation of these receptors that may underlie the sensitization of visceral nociceptors. Capsaicin-induced TPRV1 receptor-mediated changes in $[Ca^{2+}]_i$ may represent a level of DRG activation to noxious cutaneous stimulation while ATP-induced changes in $[Ca^{2+}]_i$ may reflect the level of DRG neuron sensitization to noxious visceral stimuli since ATP is released by noxious stimuli and tissue damage near the primary afferent nerve terminals (Burnstock 2001).

Most of the published reports about sex and hormone-related differences in pain have addressed the modulatory effect of E2 on central nervous system   mechanisms of nociception (Aloisi *et al.* 2000). Recent studies demonstrate that E2 has a significant role in modulating viscerosensitivity, indicating that E2-induced alterations in sensory processing may underlie sex-based differences in functional pain syndromes (Al-Chaer and Traub 2002). However, reports of E2 modulation of visceral and somatic nociceptive sensitivity are inconsistent. For example, elevated E2 levels have been reported to increase the threshold to cutaneous stimuli but decrease the percentage of escape responses to ureteral calculosis (Bradshaw and Berkley 2002). Additionally, nociceptive sensitivity increases when E2 levels are elevated (Holdcroft 2000; Bereiter 2001). Indeed in most clinical studies, women report more severe pain levels, more frequent pain and longer duration of pain than men. To help resolve these inconsistencies we propose to study E2 actions on the primary afferents.

Primary DRG neurons culture has been a useful model system for investigating sensory physiology and putative nociceptive signaling (Chaban *et al.* 2003). ATP-induced intracellular calcium concentration ($[Ca^{2+}]_i$) transients in cultured DRG neurons have been used to model the response of nociceptors to painful stimuli. In our laboratory we showed that E2, acting at the level of the plasma membrane, attenuates both ATP -induced $[Ca^{2+}]_i$ and capsaicin- induced $[Ca^{2+}]_i$ influx and that the expression of both P2X3 and TRPV1 depend on the expression of both ERs. Within the context of our hypothesis visceral nociception and nociceptor sensitization appear to be regulated by P2X3 and TRPV1. Estrogen attenuates DRG neurons response to ATP and capsaicin suggesting that visceral afferent nociceptors can be modulated by sex steroids at a new site at the level of primary afferent neurons. Our data suggest that E2 by itself appears to be anti-nociceptive but interferes with anti-nociceptive actions of other pain-modulating drugs (such as opioids). Thus, E2 acting on primary afferent nociceptors modulates the response to pro- and anti-nociceptive signals. Within the context of our cross-sensitization hypothesis, inflammation sensitizes non-inflamed viscera that are innervated by the same DRG and/or cross-sensitization occurs as a result of intra-DRG release of sensitizing mediators such as ATP or substance P in the DRG (Matsuka *et al.* 2001; Chaban 2008; Chaban 2010).

Lumbosacral DRG neurons (levels L6-S1) from wild type mice (WT) express estrogen receptors (ERα and ERβ), purinergic P2X3, vanilloid TRPV1, SP and methabotropic glutamate ($mGluR_{2/3}$) receptors. In our recent studies we also tested the difference in how somatic and visceral afferents are modulated by E2. Both short-term and long-term exposure to E2 significantly decreased the ATP and capsaicin-induced increase in $[Ca^{2+}]_i$.

2. Materials and methods

2.1 Animals

We have used 6~8 week female C57BL/6J, B6.129P2-Esr1[tm1Ksk]/J, and B6.129P2-Esr2[tm1Unc]/J mice were obtained the Jackson Laboratory (Bar Harbor, ME, USA). Upon arrival, mice were group housed in microisolator caging and maintained on a 12-h light/dark cycle in a temperature-controlled environment with access to food and water ad libitum. To test whether estrogen receptor α (ERα) or estrogen receptor β (ERβ) are involved in estradiol (E2)-induced modification of $[Ca^{2+}]_i$ Wile type, estrogen receptor alpha knock-out (ERαKO) and estrogen receptor beta knock-out (ERβKO) mice will be used. The wild type, ERαKO and ERβKO mice will be obtained from the supplier and allowed to recover for two weeks. These studies were carried out in accordance with the guidelines of the Institutional Animal

Care and Use committee at the University of California and the NIH Guide for the Care and Use of Laboratory Animals.

2.2 Animal breeding

Experiments were performed on age-matched (8–10 wk old) heterozygous mutant mice lacking the gene male (ERα−/−) and female (ERα−/−) for ERα (ERα−/−), and the deficiency ERβ (ERβ−/−) mice were bred into heterozygous mutant female mice (ERβ−/−) and homozygous male mutant mice (ERβ−/−) (Jackson Laboratory, Bar Harbor, ME, USA). Mice were housed in climate-controlled rooms, and standard rodent chow and water were available *ad libitum* and were housed in accordance with the NIH Guide for the Care and Use of Laboratory Animals

2.3 Primary culture of DRG neurons

The isolation procedure and primary culture of mouse lumbosacral DRG has been published in detail (Chaban, Mayer et al. 2003). DRG tissues were obtained from c57/black 6J (The Jackson Laboratory; 30 g), ERαKO and ERβKO (Taconic; 20 g) transgenic types. Briefly, lumbosacral adult DRGs (level L1-S1) from Wt, ERαKO and ERβKO mice will be collected under sterile technique and placed in ice-cold medium Dulbecco's Modified Eagle's Medium (DMEM; Sigma Chemical Co., St. Louis, MO). Adhering fat and connective tissue will be removed and each DRG will be minced with scissors and place immediately in a medium consisting of 5 ml of DMEM containing 0.5 mg/ml of trypsin (Sigma, type III), 1 mg/ml of collagenase (Sigma, type IA) and 0.1 mg/ml of DNAase (Sigma, type III) and kept at 37°C for 30 minutes with agitation. After dissociation of the cell ganglia, soybean trypsin inhibitor (Sigma, type III) will be used to terminate cell dissociation. Cell suspension will be centrifuged for one minute at 1000 rpm and the cell pellet will be resuspended in DMEM supplemented with 5% fetal bovine serum, 2 mM glutamine-penicillin-streptomycin mixture, 1 µg/ml DNAase and 5 ng/ml NGF (Sigma). Cells will be plated on Matrigel® (Invitrogen)-coated 15-mm coverslips (Collaborative Research Co., Bedford, PA) and kept at 37° C in 5% CO_2 incubator for 24 hrs, given fresh media and maintained in primary culture until used for experimental procedures.

2.4 Western blot analysis

The expressions of TRPV1 and of P2X3 receptors in L1~S1 DRGs were studied by using Western blot analyses. Tissues from wild type (C57BL/6J), ERαKO, and ERβKO mice were quick frozen in tubes on dry ice during collection. L1~S1 DRG were combined, homogenized by mechanical disruption in ice-cold RIPA buffer plus protease inhibitors and incubated on ice for 30 minutes. Homogenates were then spun at 5000 g for 15 minutes and supernatants collected. Total protein was determined on the supernatants using the BCA microtiter method (Pierce, Rockford, Ill., USA). Samples containing equal amounts of protein (40µg) were electrophoresed under denaturing conditions using Novex Mini-cell system (San Diego, Calif., USA) and reagents (NuPage 4–12% Bis-Tris gel and MOPS running buffer). After electrophoretic transfer onto nitrocellulose membrane using the same system, the membrane was blocked with 5% non-fat dry milk (NFDM) in 25 mM TRIS buffered saline, pH 7.2, plus Tween 20 (TBST) for 1 hour at room temperature, followed by incubation with polyclonal rabbit antibody against TRPV1-N terminus (1:1000, Neuromics) and P2X3 receptor (1:1000, Neuromics) for overnight at 4°C. The membrane was then washed in TBST plus NFDM, and incubated with secondary antibody, HRP conjugated and rabbit IgG (Santa Cruz Biotechnology) at 1:5,000 in the same buffer for 2 hours at room temperature. Following a final wash in TBST without NFDM, the membrane was incubated with ECL+ (Amersham, Arlington Heights, Ill., USA) substrate for HRP. Membranes were probed with primary antibody and corresponding secondary antibodies, signals were scanned and quantified by Image J version 1.28U and NIH Image 1.60 scan software. Following enhanced chemiluminescence (ECL) detection of proteins, the membranes were stripped and rehybridized with β-actin antibody as a loading control. At least three independent cell preparations were used.

2.5 Immunohistochemistry (IHC)

DRG tissues were obtained from C57/black 6J (The Jackson Laboratory; 30 g), ERαKO and ERβKO (Taconic; 20 g) transgenic types. Following decapitation, DRG from bilateral spinal levels L1-S2 were removed and fixed in 4% paraformaldehyde for overnight at 4°C, according to procedures approved by National Institutes of Health policy on Humane Care and Use of Laboratory Animals. DRGs were rinsed in Delbecco's Phosphate Buffered Saline (DPBS) before cryoprotection in sucrose (20%, 4°C) for two days, after which excess liquid was removed. DRG were quick snap frozen in 2-methylbutane, and store them at -70°C. Each DRG was mounted in Tissue-Tek® OCT embedding medium (Sakura Finetek), and sectioned at -20°C in a MICROM H505E cryostat. Sections were cut at 20μm and store 4°C until required. Sections of DRGs were collected in PBS. Endogenous tissue peroxidase activity was quenched by soaking the sections for 10 min in 3% hydrogen peroxide solution in 0.01 M PBS. The specimens were washed and then treated for 60 min in blocking solution, 0.01 M PBS containing 0.5% Triton X-100 and 1% normal donkey serum (NDS) at room temperature. They were processed for wild type (n=4), ERαKO (n=4), or ERβKO (n=4) immunohistochemistry by the free floating method using polyclonal rabbit TRPV1 antibody (1:50000, Neuromics) or P2X3 receptor antibody (1:15000, Neuromics) for overnight at 4°C, washed in 0.01 M phosphate-buffered saline (PBS) and 0.01M Tris Buffered Saline (TBS), followed by incubation in solutions of donkey anti-rabbit fluorophore-conjugated secondary antibodies (1:200, Invitrogen) in 0.01M Tris Buffered Saline (TBS) for 3 hours at room temperature. Cells showing no apparent or only faint membrane/intracellular labeling were considered to be negative for TRPV1 or P2X3. TRPV1-positive cells included those with strong plasma membrane labeling that formed a discernible clustered pattern, and those with strong intracellular labeling that formed a punctuate pattern. Some neurons showed both strong plasma membrane and intracellular labeling. P2X3-positive neurons showed diffuse membrane/intracellular labeling. Mounted sections were air dried and coverslipped with Aqua Poly Mount (Polisciences, Warrington, PA). Images from at least three sections in each level were taken using Leica DMLB M130X microscope. The total numbers of DRG neurons expressing TRPV1 and P2X3 were counted. TRPV1- or P2X3-positive neurons were categorized according to their labeling patterns and were expressed as a percentage of the total number of TRPV1- or P2X3-positive cells. Immunohistochemical signal percent was measured by computerized image analysis (Image Pro-Plus, Media Cybernetics, Silver Spring, MD, USA).

2.6 [Ca²⁺]ᵢ fluorescence imaging

Ca²⁺ fluorescence imaging was carried out as previously described (Gschossmann et al. 2000, Chaban et al. 2001). DRG neurons were loaded with fluorescent dye Fura-2 AM (Invitrogen) for 45 min at 37°C in HBSS supplemented with 20 mM HEPES, pH 7.4. The coverslips will be mounted on a fast-perfusion chamber P-4 (World Precision Instrument) and placed on a stage of Olympus IX51 inverted microscope. Observations were made at room temperature (20-23°C) with 20X UApo/340 objective. A fast superfusion system will be used to perfuse the cells with HBSS and rapidly apply E2 and other chemicals. Fluorescence intensity at 505 nm with excitation at 334 nm and 380 nm was captured as digital images (sampling rates of 0.1-2 s). Regions of interest were identified within the soma or neuritis from which quantitative measurements will be made by re-analysis of stored image sequences using Slidebook® Digital Microscopy software. $[Ca^{2+}]_i$ was determined by ratiometric method of Fura-2 fluorescence from calibration of series of buffered Ca^{2+} standards. We applied E2 acutely for five minutes onto the experimental chamber or the culture medium for 48 hours to study the prolonged effect of E2. Repeated applications of drugs were achieved by superfusion in a rapid mixing chamber into individual neurons for specific intervals (100-500 ms). Cells were perfused with experimental media (2 ml/min) using a Rainin® peristaltic pump.

2.7 Retrograde labeling

DRG neurons innervating viscera were identified by retrograde labeling. Briefly, mice were anesthetized with isoflurane. For colonic afferents, the descending colon was exposed and Fluorogold (5% solution in PBS; Molecular Probes, Eugene, OR) was injected into the intestinal muscle wall (10 µl injections of into five to six different sites) using a Hamilton syringe (Hamilton Co., Reno, NV) with a 26-gauge needle. In another experiments we used uterus-specific DRG neurons in which tetramethylrhodamine (TMR) dye was injected in the uterus. Injection sites were carefully swabbed, the colon and uterus were extensively rinsed with 0.9% sodium chloride solution and sealed with New Skin to prevent dye leakage. The abdomen was sutured and the animals monitored for signs of pain or discomfort during the survival period. All animals were allowed to survive one week to allow for maximal transport of retrograde markers and housed in groups of two under 12/12 hours light cycle with food and water available *ad libitum*.

2.8 Statistical analysis

The amplitude of $[Ca^{2+}]_i$ response represents the difference between baseline concentration and the transient peak response to drug stimulation. Significant differences in response to chemical stimulation will be obtained by comparing $[Ca^{2+}]_i$ increases during the first stimulation with the second. A cell will be judged responsive if E2 inhibits the second $[Ca^{2+}]_i$ transient by >30% of the first. This criterion was empirically derived in preliminary experiments. All of the data are expressed as the mean ± SEM. Statistical analysis was performed using Statistical Package for the Social Sciences 12.0 (SPSS, Chicago, IL, USA). To assess the significance among different groups, data were analyzed with one-way ANOVA followed by Schéffe post hoc test. A $P < 0.05$ was considered statistically significant.

3. Results

3.1 Role of P2X3 receptors in estrogen-induced nociceptive signaling in sensory neurons

P2X3 and TRPV1 receptors expression were examined by western blot analysis of lysates from wild type, ERαKO, and ERβKO DRG tissues using a P2X3 specific primary antiserum (Fig.1 (a)). An intense band representing a ~64 kDa protein (P2X$_3$) and a ~130 kDa (TRPV1) was seen in DRG lysates from wild type animals. There was a dramatic decrease in intensity of this band using lysates made from the both knock out DRG tissues when compared with wild type control animals (>4 fold decrease of control Fig.1). When the density in the control group was standardized to 1.0, the average densities were 0.172 ± 0.08 of ERαKO and 0.262 ± 0.10 of ERβKO in P2X3 receptors, and 0.59 ± 0.06 of ERαKO and 0.391 ± 0.04 of ERβKO in TRPV1 receptors, suggesting that both P2X3 and TRPV1 protein decreased in DRG, $P<0.05$, n=10.

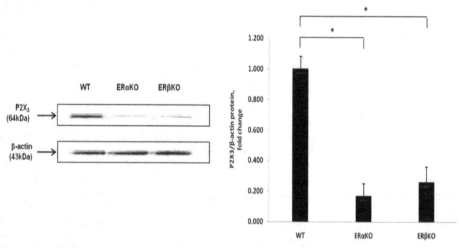

Fig. 1. Western blot analysis of DRG lysates shows reduced expression of P2X3 and TRPV1 in both knock-out mice.

Our study show that nociceptive capsaicin-sensitive TRPV1 receptors and ATP-sensitive P2X3 receptors express in DRG neurons. DRGs section were immunostained with primary antibodies against P2X3 and TRPV1. Neuronal profiles from each four mouse with ERαKO, ERβKO as well as wild type mice were quantified for each fluorescent probe. Both P2X3 and TRPV1 receptors present in DRGs (Fig. 2).

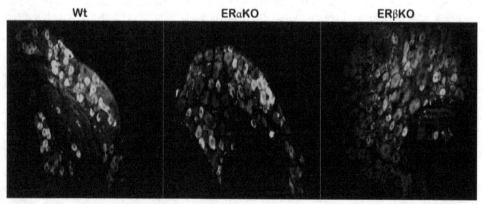

Fig. 2. Expression of P2X3 receptors in DRG neurons from wild type, ERαKO, and ERβKO *in vivo*

In our next experiments we evaluated P2X3 receptors modulation by ATP and E2 in sensory neurons. DRG neurons were loaded with fluorescent dye Fura-2 AM for one hour at 37°C in HBSS supplemented with 20 mM HEPES, pH 7.4. The coverslips were placed on a stage of Olympus IX51 inverted microscope. A fast superfusion system was used to perfuse the cells with HBSS and rapidly apply E_2 and other chemicals. Fluorescence intensity was captured as digital images (sampling rates of 0.1- 2s). Regions of interest were identified within the soma from which quantitative measurements were made by re-analysis of stored image sequences using Slidebook® Digital Microscopy software. [Ca^{2+}]$_i$ was determined by ratiometric method.

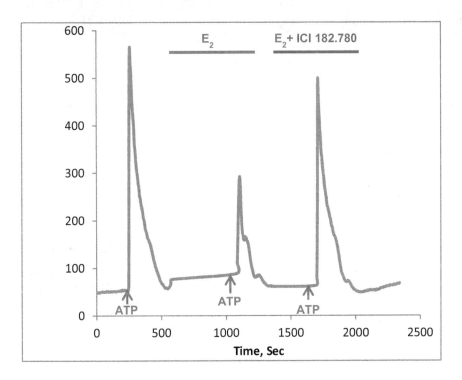

Fig. 3. 17 β-Estradiol (E2) significantly reduced ATP-induced [Ca^{2+}]$_i$ signaling *in vitro*. This effect was blocked by ER antagonist ICI 182 780

3.2 Role of TRPV1 receptors in estrogen-induced nociceptive signaling in sensory neurons

We found that nociceptive (small diameter) DRG neurons also express capsaicin-sensitive vanilloid (TRPV1) receptors. TRPV1positive neurons were categorized according to their labeling patterns and were expressed as a percentage of the total number of TRPV1 -positive cells. Immunohistochemical signal from ERαKO, ERβKO and WT mice was measured by computerized image analysis (Fig. 4)

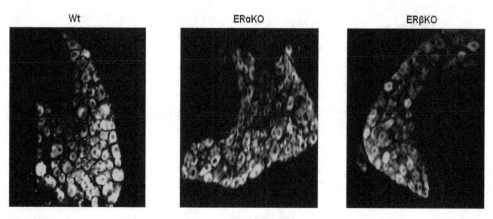

Fig. 4. Expression of TRPV1 receptors in dorsal root ganglion neurons from Wt, ERαKO, and ERβKO *in vivo*.

Capsaicin-induced TPRV1 receptor-mediated changes in $[Ca^{2+}]_i$ may represent a level of DRG activation to noxious cutaneous stimulation while ATP-induced changes in $[Ca^{2+}]_i$ may reflect the level of DRG neuron sensitization to noxious visceral stimuli since ATP is released by noxious stimuli and tissue damage near the primary afferent nerve terminals . In the view of this fact, TRPV1 receptor expression and activity might be considered as markers for a specific subtype of sensory neurons, and their activation by exogenous stimuli (e.g. capsaicin) could be a useful tool to exam the possible modulatory effects of pain-related substances.

3.3 Primary afferent sensory neurons receive input from different visceral organs

An important test of our hypothesis will be to establish that E2 modulates visceral afferents. A corollary of that hypothesis was that cutaneous pain may be differently modulated compared with visceral pain. We have proposed that E2 preferentially acts on visceral afferents to modulate the nociception. In a series of experiments using retrograde tract

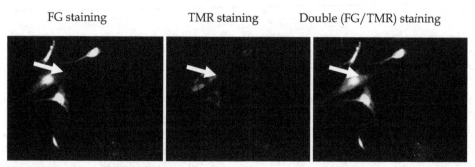

Fig. 5. Identification of colon-specific (with FG), uterus-specific (with TMR) and DRG receiving input from both organs *in vitro*

tracing we identified cutaneous and visceral afferent neurons *in vivo and in vitro*. We also found a subset of DRG neurons which innervate both visceral organs: uterus and colon.

4. Conclusion

Endometriosis is one of the most common benign gynecological diseases, characterized by the presence of endometrial tissue outside the uterine cavity, most commonly implanted over visceral and peritoneal surfaces within the female pelvis. Clinical studies have shown that it may occur in up to 10-15% of women of reproductive age. Symptoms of endometriosis are usually associated with pelvic pain, including recurrent painful periods, painful intercourse, and painful defecation during menstruation, chronic lower abdominal pain and hypersensitivity. Unfortunately, understanding of the mechanisms of endometriosis-associated pain and its management in women is currently insufficient. Studies have shown possible mechanisms of chronic pelvic pain associated with endometriosis could be due to persistent nociceptive input from endometrial tissues that lead to peripheral and central sensitisation resulting in increased responsiveness of dorsal root ganglion and dorsal horn neurons. Indeed, recent studies in human and animals have shown that peritoneal endometrial lesions are richly innervated by Aδ and C sensory nerve fibers, which positively stained by substance P or calcitonin gene-related peptide.

Several lines of evidence indicated that there is a close relationship between nerve fiber density and endometriosis-associated pain. There is a significant increase in nerve fiber density in women with endometriosis who reported pelvic pain, suggesting these nerve fibers may play an important role in the mechanisms of pain generation. Accumulating literatures described that SP presents in the myometrium and is involved in the inflammatory and pain responses, suggesting a possible role of SP nerve fibers in the generation of pain related to endometriosis. SP, which is synthesized and contained in 20–30% of DRG neurons, is involved in the transmission of nociceptive information to the central nerve system. SP is contained primarily in, and co-released from, small-diameter primary afferent fibers on noxious stimulation. Activation of nociceptive C and Aδ primary afferent fibers by electrical, chemical, or mechanical stimulation has been reported to release SP. Visceral nociceptive C-fibers can be activated by SP, representing an endogenous system regulating inflammatory, immune responses, and visceral hypersensitivity. SP afferent fibers play an important role in the pathogenesis of visceral hyperalgesia, suggesting critical role of SP in regulation of pelvic nociception associated with endometriosis. ATP is a peripheral mediator of pain which contributes to the activation of sensory afferents by activating ATP receptors following inflammation or nerve injury. It may correlate with SP release and play an important role in modulating nociception in primary sensory neurons. Local injections of ATP and ATP analogs to the rat hindpaw elicit spontaneous pain behaviors, hyperalgesia and allodynia which can be augmented by inflammation, indicating ATP might be involved in visceral hyperalgesia associated with endometriosis. Although these findings reveal the greater abundance of primary sensory nerve fibers clearly present within the peritoneal endometrial lesions in patients diagnosed with endometriosis, and these nerve fibers may play an important role in pain generation associated with endometriosis, pain mechanisms associated with endometriosis are still not well known, and the role of these primary sensory nerve fibers has not been specifically determined.

Our data support the idea that E2 modulates nociceptive responses in pelvic pain syndromes such as endometriosis, however, whether E_2 is pro- or anti-nociceptive remains unresolved. Within the context of our hypothesis visceral nociception and nociceptor sensitization appear to be regulated by P2X3 and TRPV1. E2 modulates DRG neurons response to ATP and capsaicin suggesting that visceral afferent nociceptors are modulated by E2 in the DRG. The DRG is an important site of visceral afferent convergence and cross-sensitization. We have demonstrated that 17-β estradiol (E2), the most common form of estrogen act on functional properties of P2X3 and TRPV1 receptors in DRG neurons *in vitro*. DRG neurons from Wt and knock-out mice responded to P2X3 and TRPV1 activation. We also studied the long-term (chronic) exposure to E2 on sensory neurons that mimics the temporal pattern of circulating E2 levels in cycling female rodents which is equivalent to an E2 primal action on animal reproductive behavior. The localization of ER in DRG neurons and the attenuation of ATP/capsaicin- induce $[Ca^{2+}]_i$ strongly suggest that E2 modulates visceral pain processing peripherally. Moreover, E2 appears to have different actions on nociceptive signaling depending on the input. Adult DRG neurons in short-term culture retain the expression of receptors (P2X and TRPV1) which mediate the response to putative nociceptive signals. They continue to respond to ER agonists mimicking *in vivo* activation. An important advantage is that these neurons can be studied apart from endogenous signals. Our data clearly showed the new role of nociceptors in pathophysiological aspects of chronic pelvic pain and potential way of designing future therapies.

5. References

Al-Chaer, E. D. and R. J. Traub (2002). "Biological basis of visceral pain: recent developments." Pain 96(3): 221-225.

Aloisi, A. M., I. Ceccarelli, et al. (2000). "Gonadectomy and persistent pain differently affect hippocampal c-Fos expression in male and female rats." Neurosci Lett 281(1): 29-32.

Bereiter, D. A. (2001). "Sex differences in brainstem neural activation after injury to the TMJ region." Cells Tissues Organs 169(3): 226-237.

Berkley, K. J., A. Cason, et al. (2001). "Vaginal hyperalgesia in a rat model of endometriosis." Neurosci Lett 306(3): 185-188.

Berkley, K. J., A. J. Rapkin, et al. (2005). "The pains of endometriosis." Science 308(5728): 1587-1589.

Bradshaw, H. B. and K. J. Berkley (2002). "Estrogen replacement reverses ovariectomy-induced vaginal hyperalgesia in the rat." Maturitas 41(2): 157-165.

Burnstock, G. (2000). "P2X receptors in sensory neurones." Br J Anaesth 84(4): 476-488.

Burnstock, G. (2001). "Purine-mediated signalling in pain and visceral perception." Trends Pharmacol Sci 22(4): 182-188.

Chaban, V. V. (2008). "Visceral sensory neurons that innervate both uterus and colon express nociceptive TRPv1 and P2X3 receptors in rats." Ethn Dis 18(2 Suppl 2): S2-20-24.

Chaban, V. V. (2010). "Peripheral sensitization of sensory neurons." Ethn Dis 20(1 Suppl 1): S1-3-6.

Chaban, V. V., E. A. Mayer, et al. (2003). "Estradiol inhibits ATP-induced intracellular calcium concentration increase in dorsal root ganglia neurons." Neuroscience 118(4): 941-948.

Chang, L. and M. M. Heitkemper (2002). "Gender differences in irritable bowel syndrome." Gastroenterology 123(5): 1686-1701.

Davis, J. B., J. Gray, et al. (2000). "Vanilloid receptor-1 is essential for inflammatory thermal hyperalgesia." Nature 405(6783): 183-187.

Dunn, P. M., Y. Zhong, et al. (2001). "P2X receptors in peripheral neurons." Prog Neurobiol 65(2): 107-134.

Giamberardino, M. A., R. Costantini, et al. (2010). "Viscero-visceral hyperalgesia: characterization in different clinical models." Pain 151(2): 307-322.

Gschossmann, J. M., V. V. Chaban, et al. (2000). "Mechanical activation of dorsal root ganglion cells in vitro: comparison with capsaicin and modulation by kappa-opioids." Brain Res 856(1-2): 101-110.

Holdcroft, A. (2000). "Hormones and the gut." Br J Anaesth 85(1): 58-68.

Koshimizu, T. A., F. Van Goor, et al. (2000). "Characterization of calcium signaling by purinergic receptor-channels expressed in excitable cells." Mol Pharmacol 58(5): 936-945.

Lee, D. Y., Y. G. Chai, et al. (2002). "17Beta-estradiol inhibits high-voltage-activated calcium channel currents in rat sensory neurons via a non-genomic mechanism." Life Sci 70(17): 2047-2059.

Malykhina, A. P. (2007). "Neural mechanisms of pelvic organ cross-sensitization." Neuroscience 149(3): 660-672.

Matsuka, Y., J. K. Neubert, et al. (2001). "Concurrent release of ATP and substance P within guinea pig trigeminal ganglia in vivo." Brain Res 915(2): 248-255.

Mayer, E. A., B. D. Naliboff, et al. (2001). "Basic pathophysiologic mechanisms in irritable bowel syndrome." Dig Dis 19(3): 212-218.

Micevych, P. E., V. V. Chaban, et al. (2002). "Oestrogen modulates cholecystokinin: opioid interactions in the nervous system." Pharmacology & toxicology 91: 387-397.

Micevych, P. E. and K. Sinchak (2001). "Estrogen and endogenous opioids regulate CCK in reproductive circuits." Peptides 22: 1235-1244.

Nadal, A., M. Diaz, et al. (2001). "The estrogen trinity: membrane, cytosolic, and nuclear effects." News Physiol Sci 16: 251-255.

Papka, R. E. and M. Storey-Workley (2002). "Estrogen receptor-alpha and -beta coexist in a subpopulation of sensory neurons of female rat dorsal root ganglia." Neurosci Lett 319(2): 71-74.

Petruska, J. C., J. Napaporn, et al. (2000). "Subclassified acutely dissociated cells of rat DRG: histochemistry and patterns of capsaicin-, proton-, and ATP-activated currents." J Neurophysiol 84(5): 2365-2379.

Pezzone, M. A., R. Liang, et al. (2005). "A model of neural cross-talk and irritation in the pelvis: implications for the overlap of chronic pelvic pain disorders." Gastroenterology 128(7): 1953-1964.

Zimmermann, M. (2001). "Pathobiology of neuropathic pain." Eur J Pharmacol 429(1-3): 23-37.

2

Pathomechanism of Infertility in Endometriosis

Hendi Hendarto
Dept. of Obstetric & Gynecology Faculty of Medicine,
University of Airlangga / Dr. Soetomo Hospital, Surabaya,
Indonesia

1. Introduction

Endometriosis is defined as the presence of endometrial-like tissue outside the uterus, which induces a chronic, inflammatory reaction (Kennedy *et al.*, 2005). Infertility is one of clinical manifestation of endometriosis showed by the difference of fecundity. At our tertiary hosital pelvic endometriosis is frequently found in infertile women: 23,8 % (1987), 37,2 % (1993) and 50 % (2002) cases of diagnostic laparoscopy (Samsulhadi, 2002).

An association between endometriosis and infertility has repeatedly been reported in the literature, but an absolute cause-effect relationship has not yet been confirmed. The controversy regarding whether endometriosis is a cause of infertility or an incidental finding is ongoing (ASRM, 2006; Gupta *et al.*, 2008). Many theories of endometriosis which may impair fertility have been suggested during the years, and new hypotheses and approaches to the problem have arisen with the application of assisted reproduction techniques (Garrido *et al.*, 2002). Data on the impact of endometriosis on the results of in-vitro fertilization and embryo transfer (IVF-ET) treatment are not consistent. Several theories have been proposed to identify the pathomechanism of infertility in endometriosis. None of these theories can completely explain these association. Based on many reports the possible mechanisms that could cause infertility in endometriosis are pelvic adhesion and endometrioma and also excess production of inflammatory factors in micro environment that both play a role in alteration fertility function. Severe endometriosis is associated with pelvic adhesions leading to a possible mechanic or anatomic disturbance of fertility, in the other hand a mild stage may have a direct and indirect negative effect on folliculogenesis, oocyte development, sperm function, embryogenesis, and endometrium receptivity (Barnhart *et al.*, 2002). Our aim in the present review is to describe an update on several approaches of the pathomechanism of infertility in endometriosis, based on its impact on a number of pathologic conditions, such as: pelvic adhesion and endometrioma, abnormal folliculogenesis and impaired oocyte function, altered sperm function, reduced embryo quality, and impaired endometrium receptivity.

2. Pelvic adhesion and endometrioma

The mechanisms by which endometriosis impairs fertility have not been completely determined but are likely varied. Ovarian involvement and adhesion that block tubal motility and pick-up of the egg could be a main causative of mechanical interference on fertility especially in severe endometriosis due to a possible mechanic or anatomic disturbance such as extensive pelvic adhesions. Pelvic endometriosis, the most common form of the disease, could be associated with increased secretion of pro-inflammatory cytokines, impaired cell-mediated immunity and neo-angiogenesis. Barnhart *et al.* (2002) found that compared with women with mild endometriosis, women with severe endometriosis have a statistically significantly lower pregnancy rate and implantation rate, have fewer oocytes obtained at ovarian retrieval, and have a lower peak estradiol concentration (Barnhart *et al.*, 2002).

Adhesion formation involves three important components: 1) acute inflammatory response, 2) fribinolysis, and 3) metalloproteinases and their tissue inhibitors. Celluler mediators within the peritoneal fluid can potentially modulate inflammatory responses over a large surface area due to the liquid nature of the peritoneal fluid. There are three important pro-inflammatory cytokines involved in adhesion formation: interleukine (IL)-1, IL-6 and Tumor Necrosis Factor (TNF)-α (Cheong *et al.*, 2002). Endometriosis is associated with signs of pelvic peritoneal inflammation including increased volume of peritoneal fluid, increased concentration of peritoneal fluid macrophages, and increased peritoneal fluid concentrations of IL-6, IL-8, TNF-α and other cytokines and growth factors. Indeed, these cytokines have been reported to increase the endometrial–peritoneal adhesion *in vitro* (D'Hooghe and Debrock, 2002). Pelvic adhesion secondary to endometriosis is the most accepted reason for infertility, presumably via dysfunction of the fallopian tube or ovary. Inflammatory cytokines, IL-6, IL- 8 and TNF-α produced by endometrial cells probably contribute to the adhesion process. IL-8 has been shown to stimulate the adhesion of endometrial cells to fibronectin. TNF-α has also been reported to promote endometrial stromal cell proliferation *in vitro* and endometrial stromal cell adhesion to extracellular matrix components (Garcia-Velasco and Arici, 1999). These pelvic adhesion inhibits ovum capture after ovulation.

Cysts of endometriosis (endometriomas) may become adherent to the uterus, bowel or pelvic side wall. Any of these anatomic distortions can result in infertility. The presence of an ovarian endometrioma greater than 1 cm in diameter is classified as stage III (moderate) or more in the revised American Society for Reproductive Medicine (ASRM) classification of endometriosis, but unfortunately, the staging system does not correlate well with a woman's chance of conception following therapy (ASRM, 2006). The impact of an ovarian endometrioma on infertility remains controversial, despite the number of studies that have been performed. Suzuki *et al* (2005) found that endometriosis, even after diagnostic laparoscopy with treatment when necessary, clearly affects the number of oocytes as well as the number of transferred embryos but not embryo quality and the related parameters of pregnancy, as indicated by the fertilization rate, embryo quality, implantation rate, pregnancy rate, and live birth rate, irrespective of the presence of an ovarian endometrioma (Suzuki *et al*, 2005). Nakahara (1998) found that the proportion of apoptotic bodies in the membrana granulosa cells and the cumulus cells from patients with endometrioma is significantly higher than that in patients without endometrioma. Based on these studies endometrioma prove the existence of a more advance stage of endometriosis than the non existence of endometrioma. The existence of endometrioma is considered one of the indicators of endometriosis in the ovary due to the increase of the apoptosis in the follicle and gave, in turn, the follicle an atretic status. Consequently, patients with endometriosis with endometrioma had smaller numbers of follicles developed, oocytes harvested, and mature oocytes (Nakahara *et al*, 1998).

In women with endometriosis, pelvic adhesions contain estrogen and progesterone receptors, and produce basic fibroblastic growth factor and vascular endothelial growth factor, implying a regulation of pelvic adhesion formation by steroid hormone. Zang (2010) found that both the percentage and the density of protein gene product (PGP) 9.5-positive nerve fibres in ovarian endometriotic lesions were significantly higher in women with ovarian endometriosis who had pelvic adhesions than in those women with ovarian endometriosis and no pelvic adhesions (Zang et al., 2010). It is suggested that ovarian endometriotic lesions may be innervated through mediating effects of peritoneal inflammatory cytokines and growth factors including IL-1, IL-6 and TNF-a, in women with pelvic adhesions, thus leading to an increase of nerve fibres in ovarian endometriotic lesions in women with ovarian endometriosis (Zang *et al.*, 2010).

3. Abnormal folliculogenesis and impaired oocyte function

Infertility associated with the advanced stages of endometriosis may be explained by pelvic adhesion and endometrioma as described above. The mechanism of infertility associated with endometriosis without adhesion and endometrioma, such as minimal or mild endometriosis as well as the negative impact of all stages of the disease on infertility is poorly understood. Many possibilities have been suggested, ranging from abnormal folliculogenesis to impaired endometrium receptivity (Arici *et al.*, 1999). Peritoneal fluid, a biologic fluid present in the abdominal cavity, has been a focus of research on endometriosis because of the extent of information it potentially carries about the disease. The proximity of peritoneal fluid to endometriotic lesions shows the milieu in which the immune mediators associated with the local inflammation of endometriosis can be studied. It has been suggested that such alterations in cytokines and growth factors interfere with folliculogenesis, ovulation and fertilization (Arici *et al.*, 1999).

The local microenvironment of peritoneal fluid surrounding the endometriotic implant is immunologically dynamic and links the reproductive and immune systems. Peritoneal fluid contains a variety of free floating cells, including macrophages, mesothelial cells, lymphocytes, eosinophils and mast cells (Oral *et al.*, 1996). The peritoneal fluid of women with endometriosis have confirmed an increased number, concentration and activation of macrophages which may induce proliferation of cells that are involved in inflammation through secretion of factors such as IL- 1, IL-6, and TNF-α (Oral *et al.*, 1996a). Other studies similary found that levels of cytokines, such as, IL-6, IL-8 and TNF-α increased in the peritoneal fluid of women with endometriosis (Arici *et al.*, 1996), meanwhile endometriotic implants also secreted various cytokines including IL-1, IL-6, IL-8, TNF-α in the peritoneal cavity in patients with endometriosis (Oral *et al.*, 1996b). Cytokines, which are produced by many cell types in peritoneal fluid, play a diverse role as toxic effect in constructing the peritoneal environment that induces the development and progression of endometriosis and endometriosis-associated infertility (Harada *et al.*, 2001).

Peritoneal fluid bathed the ovaries, hypothetically the inflammatory components in peritoneal fluid in women with endometriosis might diffuse into the ovarian follicles, or by paracrine mechanisms (Carlberg *et al.*, 2000) impair the granulosa cell function, oocyte maturation and folliculogenesis. Folliculogenesis is growth and development process of ovarian follicle consist of oocyte, granulosa and theca cells might result in mature and fertilizable oocyte (Rajkovic, 2006). The alteration of oocyte, granulosa, theca cells development and molecular follicular communication may impact on folliculogenesis. Carlberg (2000) found that granulosa cells of women with endometriosis have an up-regulated production of IL-1β, IL-6, IL-8, TNF-α which might be related to the reduced fertilization rate previously observed in endometriosis women (Carlberg *et al.*, 2000). Beside that women with endometriosis were reported having higher granulosa cell apoptosis rate and a lower percentage of G2/M phase granulosa cells compared with other group of infertile women. This result strongly suggest that the cytokines produced in endometriosis women may be responsible for the disturbance of the cell cycle in the granulosa cells as in other cells and in turn have pathogenic effects on folliculogenesis (Toya *et al.* 2000) . Nakahara (1998) found that higher incidence of apoptotic bodies correlates with a lower quality of oocytes in individual follicles. This study showed that the incidence of apoptotic bodies in membrana granulosa ovaries of patients with endometriosis undergoing the IVF-ET procedure was increased as the stage of the revised AFS classification advanced. It means that the quality of oocytes from patients with endometriosis decreases in proportion to advancing stages of the revised AFS classification and determine the degree of disturbance for folliculogenesis in the ovaries of the patients with endometriosis (Nakahara, 1998).

Our previous study postulated that apoptosis of granulosa cells caused disturbance in oocyte growth and maturation and associated with decreased growth differentiation factor-9 (GDF-9) production (Hendarto *et al.*, 2010). Oocyte-derived GDF-9 is obligatory for normal folliculogenesis and female fertility (Erickson and Shimasaki, 2001). Elvin (1999) reported that mouse GDF-9 can bind to receptors on granulosa cells, and plays multifunctional roles in oocyte-granulosa cell communication and regulation of follicular differentiation and function (Elvin *et al.*, 1999). In our study we found that the presence of GDF-9 in follicular fluid of preovulatory follicle was confirmed by western blotting analysis in a band of 53 kDa, and compared with the level in women with no endometriosis, GDF-9 level in the follicular fluid of women with severe endometriosis was lower. This might impair folliculogenesis, leading to reduced oocyte quality (Hendarto *et al.*, 2010). Our other study also comfirmed that oocyte-granulosa cell communication has already been altered showed by increasing the concentration of granulosa cell-derived kit-ligand in follicular fluid of infertile women with endometriosis (in publication process).

The cytoskeleton of metaphase II oocytes were influenced by rich pro-inflammatory factor present in peritoneal fluid of patients with endometriosis. By exposure of cryopreserved mouse oocytes to the peritoneal fluid from women with endometriosis, Mansour (2010) reported that in the endometriosis group, the cytoskeleton had a higher frequency of abnormal meiotic spindle and chromosomal misalignment, indicating severe damage compared with the control groups. The meiotic spindle plays a critical role in maintaining chromosomal organization and formation of the second polar body. Disorganization of the meiotic spindle can result in chromosomal dispersion, failure of normal fertilization, and abnormal development. Alterations of the spindle may be one of the many causes related to infertility and/or recurrent pregnancy loss in patients with endometriosis (Mansour *et al.,* 2010). Reactive oxygen species (ROS) have been detected in peritoeal fluid of endometriosis patients but are not significantly elevated compared with the control and idiopathic infertility groups (Bedaiwy *et al.,* 2002). Reactive oxygen species have detrimental effects on oocytes, they are able to diffuse and pass through cell membrane and alter most types of cellular molecule such as lipids, proteins and nucleic acids. The consequences are mitochondrial alterations, embryo cell block, ATP depletion and apoptosis (Guerin, 2001).

Based on several studies above it is proposed that pro-inflammatory factors and ROS in follicular fluid women with endometriosis may diffuse and impact autocrine-paracrine communication of ovarian follicles causing cell-cycle alteration and an increased apoptosis in granulosa cells. Beside that, the presence of pro-inflammatory factors and ROS could influence the oocyte such as abnormal meiotic spindle, chromosomal misalignment and decreased GDF-9 production. Both may impair oocyte-granulosa cell communicatin and cause abnormal folliculogenesis and, in turn, result in reduced oocyte quality. Futher studies are needed. (see figure 1)

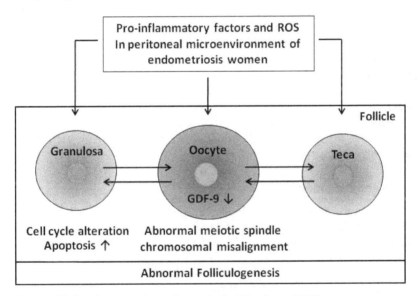

Fig. 1. Abnormal folliculogenesis in endometriosis (Hendarto, 2011)

4. Altered sperm function

Spermatozoa have to stay for a certain period of time in the female genital tract that normally favors capacitation, the ability to reach and fertilize the oocyte. The endometriosis-associated immuno-inflammatory changes in peritoneal fluid may have some adverse effects on spermatozoa (Carli *et al.,* 2007). Eisermann (1989) reported that levels of TNF-α of up to 800 U/ml in peritoneal fluid from infertile women with endometriosis higher than fertile women without endometriosis. In this concentration,

TNF-α caused a significant reduction in both progressive and total sperm motility when compared with controls group. Suggests that this may be a mechanism for the infertility observed in women with minimal endometriosis (Eisermann *et al.*, 1989). In the other study stated that the toxic effects of TNF-α could be the result of its ability to stimulate apoptosis in sperm cells through initiation of a caspase cascade. Exposing spermatozoa to pathological concentrations of TNF-α can result in significant loss of sperm function and genomic integrity. Infliximab, an TNF-α inhibitor, could potentially be used to help treat female infertility caused by endometriosis in those with elevated levels of TNF-α in their peritoneal fluid (Said *et al.*, 2005).

Another theory describing pathological effect of endometriosis on sperm function is the role of reactive oxygen species. Oxidative stress has been shown to exert toxic effects on sperm, damaging the sperm cell membrane, inducing DNA damage, and mediating sperm apoptosis (Agarwal *et al.*, 2006). Mansour (2009) found that progressive sperm DNA damage was significantly higher in samples incubated with peritoneal fluid from patients with endometriosis than those from healthy women. Spermatozoa are particularly susceptible to ROS-induced damage because their plasma membranes contain large quantities of polyunsaturated fatty acids and their cytoplasm contains low concentrations of the scavenging enzymes (Saleh *et al.*, 2002)

Reeve (2005) reported that significantly more spermatozoa bound per unit area to the ampullary epithelium of the uterine tubes taken from women with endometriosis, could potentially hinder fertilization by reducing the number of free spermatozoa in the tubal lumen that are available to take part in fertilization. Numerous studies have shown that spermatozoa that bind to the endosalpinx retain their viability, motility and fertilizing capacity longer than spermatozoa incubated alone or with other cell types. The aberrant expression of integrin in the endometrium of women with endometriosis would be speculated to increased sperm binding (Reeve *et al.*, 2005).

5. Reduced embryo quality

Use of IVF-ET as a therapeutic tool in endometriosis women with infertility could result in information about this disease and reproductive process aspects, such as folliculogenesis, fertilization, embryo development and implantation. The outcome of patients with endometriosis undergoing IVF-ET showed not only the influence of endometriosis on IVF result but also the possible pathomechanisms of infertility in endometriosis (Garrido et al., 2000). The impact of endometriosis in embryo development and quality is still on debate. Various embryo scoring system have been described to assess the developmental potential of embryos, but the most commonly used systems are the blastomeres cleavage rate, the shape and size of the blastomeres and the amount of anucleated fragment (Martynow et al., 2007)

Pellicer (1995) found a significantly reduced number of blastomeres in embryos from endometriosis patients compared with controls, and endometriosis patients had a poor IVF-ET outcome in terms of a reduced pregnancy rate per cycle, reduced pregnancy rate per transfer and reduced implantation rate per embryo replaced (Pellicer et al., 1995). Simon (1994) showed that patients who received embryos derived from endometriosis ovaries showed a significantly reduced ability to implant compared with the remaining groups (Simon et al., 1994). These result above suggest that infertility in endometriosis patients may be related to alterations within the oocyte which, in turn, result in reduced embryos quality (Pellicer et al., 1995).

Endometriosis induces an inflammatory state by activation of macrophages, releasing ROS and cytokines (Gupta *et al.*, 2008). Macrophages, cytokines and other products present in the peritoneal fluid from patients with endometriosis could be responsible for a change in the peritoneal environment that generates embryotoxic activity. Torres (2002) found embryotoxicity was increased in women with endometriosis, but there was little correlation with severity of the disease. These study also found a significant increase in embryotoxicity in the presence of high cytokine concentrations, especially with IL-6 (Torres et al., 2002). Other study by Pellicer found progesterone concentrations in follicular fluid increased with the severity of endometriosis that may be related to the release of the cytokines. The result of the study also showed that IL-6 concentration was significantly increased in follicular fluid of patients with endometriosis, whereas VEGF accumulation in follicular fluid was significantly decreased in women with endometriosis compared with controls. The increased IL-6 means that the immune system may be activated as a marker of altered follicular function that result in reduced oocyte and embryo quality. The decreased VEGF concentration needs further investigation, but in IVF, elevated VEGF concentrations have been shown to be related to good follicular vascularization and health. The study by Pellicer concluded profound differences in the follicular environment of the oocytes of women with endometriosis, compared with those of healthy patients. It may be suspected as a marker of altered follicular function that result in reduced oocyte and embryo quality.

6. Impaired endometrium receptivity

There are controversial information regarding implantation alteration in endometriosis-associated infertility. Various studies described three causative factors: an oocyte/embryo impairment, endometrial defect and altered endometrial-embryonic cross-talk (Garrido *et al.*, 2002). Implantation depends on an interaction of the trophoblast with the uterine epithelium, whereas a receptive endometrium is characterized by abundant secretory activity such as the presence of several integrins including the $\alpha v \beta 3$ integrin. Lessey (1994) reported that the majority of women with abnormal $\alpha v \beta 3$ integrin expression had endometriosis stage I or II and stated that $\alpha v \beta 3$ integrin expression could be a useful marker of mild endometriosis (Lessey *et al.*, 1994). Inconsistent result pointed by Surrey (2010) that a high prevalence of aberrant endometrial $\alpha v \beta 3$ vitronectin expression was noted in a group of infertile endometriosis patients who are IVF candidates but there were no significant differences in ongoing pregnancy or implantation rates in those patients who failed to express integrin $\alpha v \beta 3$ vitronectin who were treated with a 3-month course of a GnRH agonist before an IVF cycle in comparison to untreated controls. Endometrial $\alpha v \beta 3$ integrin expression did not predict which patients would benefit from prolonged administration of a GnRH agonist before initiation of controlled ovarian hyperstimulation for IVF (Surrey *et al.*, 2010)

The detection of pinopodes as a possible marker of receptivity in humans has been extensively studied. Pinopodes are specialized cell surface formations presumably involved in the adhesion of blastocysts to the luminal epithelium. Scanning electron microscopy in sequential endometrial biopsies showed that pinopodes formed briefly (1–2 days) and that their numbers correlate with implantation (Nikas *et al.*, 1999). Garcia-Velasco (2001) found pinopode expression in women with endometriosis did not differ from that of patients without endometriosis undergoing artificial cycles. Similarly, the clinical outcome in these women was comparable to that of the general population included in the oocyte donation program and this study stated that pinopode expression is not altered, suggesting that endometrial receptivity in women with this disease remains unaltered (Garcia-Velasco *et al.*, 2001).

Endometrial aspects and molecular studies on the receptivity status of endometrium resulted in conflicting data. Several studies suggest that an altered follicular microenvironment could be responsible for a defective folliculogenesis, and subsequently reduced oocyte/embryo quality, and in turn, result in altered embryo implantation but the debate still ongoing (Garrido *et al.*, 2002).

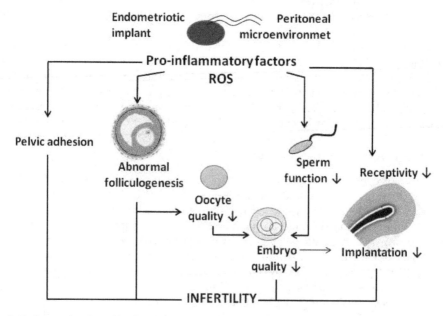

Fig. 2. Pathomechanism of infertility in endometriosis (Hendarto, 2011)

7. Summary

We have reviewed various studies with regard to the understanding of pathomechanism of infertility in endometriosis, based on its impacts on number of pathologic conditions, such as: pelvic adhesion and endometrioma, abnormal folliculogenesis and impaired oocyte function, altered sperm function, reduced embryo quality, and impaired endometrium receptivity. The controversy regarding whether endometriosis is a cause of infertility or an incidental finding is ongoing.

Based on several studies reviewed above showed that peritoneal microenvironment of women with endometriosis which contain pro-inflammatory factor and ROS is the main causative factor of the pathomechanism of infertility in endometriosis. They have a key role through autocrine-paracrine communication alteration in the mechanism of pelvic adhesion, abnormal folliculogenesis, reduced oocyte/embryo quality, reduced sperm fuction and implantaion impairment (see figure 2). We hope that the increase of our understanding on the above pathomechanism can increase our attention to the improvement of the complex management of infertility in endometriosis.

8. Acknowledgments

The author would like to thank Prof Lila Dewata and Prof Samsulhadi for their assistance in the preparation of the manuscript.

9. References

Agarwal, A., Gupta, S., & Sikkab, S. (2006). The role of free radicals and anti oxidants in reproduction. *Curr. Opin. Obstet. Gynecol.*, Vol. 18, pp. 325–332, ISSN 1040-872x.

Agarwal, A., Sharma, R.K., Nallella, K.P., & Thomas, A.J. Jr., Alvarez, J.G., Sikka, S.C. (2006). Reactive oxygen species as an independent marker of male factor infertility. *Fertil. Steril.*, Vol. 86, pp. 878–85, ISSN 1556-5653.

American Society for Reproductive Medicine (ASRM). (2006). Endometriosis and infertility. The Practice Committee of The American Society for Reproductive Medicine. *Fertil. Steril.*, Vol. 86, pp. 156-60, ISSN 1556-5653.

Arici, A., Tazuke, S.I., Attar, E., Kliman, H.J., Olive, D.L. (1996). Interleukin-8 concentration in peritoneal fluid of patients with endometriosis and modulation of interleukin-8 expression in human mesothelial cells. *Mol. Hum. Reprod.*, Vol. 2, pp. 40 –5, ISSN 1460-2407.

Barnhart, K.M., Dunsmoor, R., Su, M.S., & Coutifaris, C. (2002). Effect of endometriosis on in vitro fertilization. *Fertil. Steril.*, Vol. 77, pp. 1148-1155, ISSN 1556-5653.

Bedaiwy, M.A., Falcone, T., Sharma, R.K., Goldberg, J.M., Attaran, M., Nelson, D.R., et al. (2002). Prediction of endometriosis with serum and peritoneal fluid markers: a prospective controlled trial. Hum. Reprod., Vol. 17, pp. 426–31, ISSN 1460-2350.

Carlberg, M., Nejaty, J., Froysa, B., Guan, Y., Soder, O., & Bergqvist, A. (2000). Elevated expression of TNFα in cultured granulosa cells from women with endometriosis. *Hum. Reprod.*, Vol. 15, pp. 1250-5, ISSN 1460-2350.

Carli, C., Leclerc, P., Metz, C.N., & Akoum, A. (2007). Direct effect of macrophage migration inhibitory factor on sperm function: possible involvement in endometriosis-associated infertility. *Fertil. Steril.*, Vol. 88, pp. 1240-7, ISSN 1556-5653.

Cheong, Y.C., Shelton, J.B., Laird, S.M., Richmond, RM., Kudesia, G., Li, T.C., Ledger, W.L. (2002). IL-1, IL-6 and TNF-α concentrations in peritoneal fluid of women with pelvic adhesions. *Hum. Reprod.*, Vol. 17, pp. 69-75, ISSN 1460-2350.

D'hooghe, T.M., Debrock, S. (2002). Endometriosis, retrograde menstruation and peritoneal inflammation in women and in baboons. *Hum. Reprod. Update.*, Vol. 8, pp. 84-88, ISSN 1460-2369.

Eisermann, J., Register, K.B., Strickler, R.C., & Collins, J.L. (1989).The Effect of Tumor Necrosis Factor on Human Sperm Motility In Vifro. *J. of Andrology.*, Vol. 10, pp. 270-4, ISSN 1939-4640.

Elvin, J.A,. Clark, A.T., Wang, P., Wolfman, N.M., & Matzuk, M. (1999). Paracrine action of growth differentiation factor-9 in mammalian ovary. *Mol. Endocrinol.*, Vol. 13, pp. 1035–48, ISSN 1944-9917.

Erickson, G.F., & Shimasaki, S. (2001). The physiology of folliculogenesis: the role of novel growth factors. *Fertil. Steril.*, Vol. 76, pp. 943–9, ISSN 1556-5653.

Garcia-Velasco, J.A., Arici, A. (1999). Interleukin-8 stimulates the adhesion of endometrial stromal cells to fibronectin. *Fertil. Steril.*, Vol. 72, pp. 336-341, ISSN 1556-5653.

Garcia-Velasco, J.A., Nikas, G., Remohı´, J., Pellicer, J.A., & Simon, C. (2001). Endometrial receptivity in terms of pinopode expression is not impaired in women with endometriosis in artificially prepared cycles. *Fertil. Steril.*, Vol. 75, pp. 1231–3, ISSN 1556-5653.

Garrido, N., Navarro, J., Remohi, J., Simon, C., & Pellicer, A. (2000). Hormonal follicular environment and embryo quality in women with endometriosis. *Hum. Reprod. Updat.e*, Vol. 6, No. 1, pp. 67-74, ISSN 1460-2369.

Garrido, N., Navarro, J., Garcia-Velasco, J., Remohi, J., Pellicer, A., & Simon, C. (2002). The endometrium versus embryonic quality in endometriosis-related infertility. *Hum. Reprod. Update.*, Vol. 8, pp. 95-103, ISSN 1460-2369.

Guerin, P., El Mouatassim, S., & Menezo, Y. (2001). Oxidative stress and protection against reactive oxygen species in the pre-implantation embryo and its surroundings. *Hum. Reprod. Update.*, Vol. 7, pp. 175–89, ISSN 1460-2369

Gupta, S., Goldberg, J.M., Aziz, N., Goldberg,E., Krajcir,N., & Agarwal, A. (2008). Pathogenic mechanisms in endometriosis-associated infertility. *Fertil. Steril.*, Vol. 90, pp. 247–57, ISSN 1556-5653.

Harada, T., Iwabe, T., & Terakawa, N. (2001). Role of cytokines in endometriosis. *Fertil.Steril.*, Vol. 76, pp. 1–10, ISSN 1556-5653.

Hendarto, H., Prabowo, P., Moeloek, F.A., & Soetjipto. (2010). Growth differentiation factor 9 concentration in the follicular fluid of infertile women with endometriosis. *Fertil. Steril.*, Vol. 94, pp. 758–60, ISSN 1556-5653.

Kennedy, S., Bergqvist, A., Chapron, C., D'Hooghe, T., Dunselman, G., Greb, R., Hummelshoj, L., Prentice, A., Saridogan, E. (2005). ESHRE guideline for the diagnosis and treatment of endometriosis. *Hum. Reprod.*, Vol. 21, pp. 2698–2704, ISSN 1460-2350.

Lessey, B.A., Castelbaum, A.J., Sawin, S.W., Buck, C.A., Schinnar, R., Bilker, W., & Strom, B.L. (1994) Aberrant integrin expression in the endometrium of women with endometriosis. *J. Clin. Endocrinol. Metab.*, Vol. 79, pp. 643–649, ISSN 0021-972x

Mansour, G., Aziz, N., Sharma, R., Falcone, T., Goldberg, J., & Agarwal,A. (2009). The impact of peritoneal fluid from healthy women and from women with endometriosis on sperm DNA and its relationship to the sperm deformity index. *Fertil. Steril.*, Vol. 92, pp. 61–7, ISSN 1556-5653.

Mansour, G., Sharma, R.K., Agarwal, A., & Falcone, T. (2010). Endometriosis-induced alterations in mouse metaphase II oocyte microtubules and chromosomal alignment: a possible cause of infertility. *Fertil. Steril.*, Vol. 94, pp. 1894–9, ISSN 1556-5653.

Martynow, M.D., Jedrzejczak, P., Pawelczyk, L. (2007). Pronuclear scoring as a predictor of embryo quality in *in vitro* fertilization program. *Fol. Histo. et Cytobiol.*, Vol. 45, pp. 87-91, ISSN 0239-8508.

Nakahara, K., Saito, H., Saito, T., Ito, M., Ohta, N., Takahashi, T. et al. (1997). Ovarian fecundity in patients with endometriosis can be estimated by the incidence of apoptotic bodies. *Fertil. Steril.*, Vol. 69, pp. 931–5, ISSN 1556-5653.

Nikas, G. (1999). Pinopodes as markers of endometrial receptivity in clinical practice. *Hum. Reprod.*, Vol. 14, pp. 99 –106, ISSN 1460-2350.

Omwandho, C.O.A., Konrad, L., Halis, G.I., Oehmke, F., & Tinneberg, H.R. (2010). Role of TGF-bs in normal human endometrium and endometriosis. *Hum. Reprod.*, Vol. 25, pp. 101–109, ISSN 1460-2350.

Oral, E., Olive, D.L., & Arici, A. (1996a). The peritoneal environment in endometriosis. *Hum. Reprod. Update.*, Vol. 2, No. 5, pp. 385-398 , ISSN 1460-2369.

Oral, E., Seli, E., Bahtiyar, M., Olive, D., & Arici, A. (1996b). Growth regulated alpha expression in the peritoneal environment with endometriosis. *Obstet. Gyneco.l*, Vol. 88, pp.1050-6, ISSN 0020-7292.

Pellicer, A., Oliveira, N., Ruiz, A., Remohí, J., & Simón, C. (1995). Exploring the mechanism(s) of endometriosis-related infertility: an analysis of embryo development and implantation in assisted reproduction. *Hum. Reprod*, Vol. 10, pp. 91-97, ISSN 1460-2350.

Rajkovic, A., Pangas, S.A., & Matzuk, M.M. (2006). Follicular Development: Mouse, sheep and human models. In: *Knobil and Neill's Physiology of Reproduction*, Neill JD, pp 383-424. 3rd ed. Elsevier, ISBN: 978-0-12-515400-0, Los Angeles.

Reeve, L., Lashen, H., & Pacey, A.A. (2005). Endometriosis affects sperm–endosalpingeal interactions. *Hum. Reprod.*, Vol. 20, 448–451, ISSN 1460-2350

Said, T.M., Agarwal, A., Falcone, T., Sharma, R.K., Mohamed, A.. Bedaiwy, M.A., & Liang, L. (2005). Infliximab may reverse the toxic effects induced by tumor necrosis factor alpha in human spermatozoa: an in vitro model. *Fertil. Steril.*, Vol. 83, 1665–73, ISSN 1556-5653.

Saleh, R.A., Agarwal, A. (2002). Oxidative stress and male infertility: from research bench to clinical practice. *J. Androl.*, Vol. 23, pp. 737–752, ISSN 0196-3635.

Samsulhadi. (2002). Endometriosis: Dari biomolekuler sampai masalah klinis (Endometriosis : from biomoleculer to clinical application). *Majalah Obstetri dan Ginekologi*, Vol.10, pp. 43-50.

Simón, C., Gutiérrez, A., Vidal, A., Santos M.J dr los., Tarín J.J, Remohí, J., Pellicer, A. (1994). Outcome of patients with endometriosis in assisted reproduction: results from in-vitro fertilization and oocyte donation. *Hum. Reprod.*, Vol. 9 , pp. 725-729, ISSN 1460-2350.

Surrey, E.S., Lietz, A.K., Gustofson, R.L., Minjarez, D.A., & Schoolcraft, W.B. (2010). Does endometrial integrin expression in endometriosis patients predict enhanced in vitro fertilization cycle outcomes after prolonged GnRH agonist therapy? *Fertil. Steril.*, Vol. 93, pp. 646–51, ISSN 1556-5653.

Suzuki, T., Izumi, S., Matsubayashi, H., Awaji, H., Yoshikata, K., Makino, T. (2005). Impact of ovarian endometrioma on oocytes and pregnancy outcome in in vitro fertilization. *Fertil. Steril.*, Vol. 83, pp. 908-13, ISSN 1556-5653.

Torres, M.J.G., Acien, P., Campos, A., Velasco, I. (2002). Embryotoxicity of follicular fluid in women with endometriosis. Its relation with cytokines and lymphocytes populations. Hum. Reprod., Vol. 17, pp. 777-781, ISSN 1460-2350.

Toya, M., Saito, H., Ohta, N., Saito, T., Kaneko, T., & Hiroi, M. (2000). Moderate and severe endometriosis is associated with alterations in the cell cycle of granulosa cells in patients undergoing in vitro fertilization and embryo transfer. *Fertil. Steril.*, Vol. 73, pp. 344 –50, ISSN 1556-5653.

Zhang, X., Yao, H., Huang, X., Lu, B., Hong Xu, H., & Zhou, C. (2010). Nerve fibres in ovarian endometriotic lesions in women with ovarian endometriosis. *Hum. Reprod.*, Vol. 25, pp. 392–397, ISSN 1460-2350.

3

Endometriosis-Associated Ovarian Cancer: The Role of Oxidative Stress

Yoriko Yamashita and Shinya Toyokuni
Nagoya University Graduate School of Medicine,
Japan

1. Introduction

Recent studies indicated that oxidative stress has a causal role in the carcinogenesis of mainly two histological subtypes of ovarian cancer, namely, clear cell carcinoma and endometrioid adenocarcinoma. Because of recurrent hemorrhage in endometrial cysts, excess of reactive oxygen species are produced due to iron deposition, which results in direct genomic mutation of the epithelial cells and exaggeration of oxidative stress by stromal cells such as macrophages. In endometriosis-associated ovarian cancer, genomic mutations in specific genes such as ARID1A, p53, K-ras, PTEN, PI3CA and Met have been reported. Mechanism of carcinogenesis, especially focusing on the precise role of oxidative stress, remains to be clarified. Development of novel drugs and methods for therapy or prevention of endometriosis-associated ovarian cancer is necessary.

2. Risk of cancer development in endometriosis

Endometriosis is a common disease affecting 10 to 15% of women of reproductive age (Irving, 2011). An association between endometriosis and cancer was reported as early as the 1920s in English publications. Sampson (Sampson, 1925) proposed that endometrial carcinoma of the ovary develops from endometrial tissue, based on classic microscopic observation using several strict criteria (i.e., the coexistence of benign and malignant tissue with a shared histologic relationship in the same organ and evidence against invasion from other sites or sources). Further studies were interrupted by World War II; however, in the late 1940s and 1950s, several groups published case reports that met Sampson's criteria (Scott, 1953; Postoloff & Rodenberg, 1955). Although none of the studies demonstrated any direct evidence, the consensus of the major researchers in the field at that time was that malignant transformation or transition occurred in ovarian endometriosis.

In 1990, Heaps et al. analyzed 195 cases that mostly fulfilled Sampson's criteria (Heaps, 1990). They found that the primary endometriosis site was most frequently the ovary (78.7%), followed by various other sites such as the pelvis, rectovaginal septum, colon or rectum, or the vagina. The most frequent histologic subtype was endometrioid adenocarcinoma in either of the primary sites, ovarian (69%) or extragonadal (66%), followed by clear cell carcinoma and sarcoma in 13.5% and 11.6% of ovarian tumors, respectively, and sarcomas in 25% of extragonadal tumors. More recently, an elevated risk of ovarian cancer development in endometriosis has been shown by statistical analyses. A direct prospective study of 20,686 Swedish patients hospitalized with endometriosis between 1969 and 1983 with a mean follow-up period of 11.4 years demonstrated a standardized incidence ratio (SIR) of 1.9 and a 95% confidence interval [CI] of 1.3 to 2.8 (Brinton, 1997). Similar results were reported in a case-control study analyzing patients from the United States, in which the relative risk for ovarian cancer development in endometriosis patients was 1.7 (Ness, 2000). A nationwide case-control study of Australian patients with ovarian cancer revealed that endometriosis increased the risks of both endometrioid adenocarcinoma and clear cell carcinoma, with odds ratios of 3.0 and 2.2, respectively (Nagle, 2008). A recent retrospective study from Canada also showed a significant increase in the relative risk (rate ratio [RR], 1.6; 95% CI, 1.12 to 2.09) of ovarian cancer in patients with endometriosis (Aris, 2010). In line with these reports, a recent prospective study from Japan showed a significant and much greater elevation in the relative risk (SIR, 8.95; CI, 4.12 to 115.3) of cancer development in Japanese patients with endometrioma, or endometrial cyst of the ovary (Kobayashi, 2007). The reason for this discrepancy is unclear, but one possibility is that the endometriosis patients in the Japanese study included only those with clinically detectable ovarian endometrial cysts. It is also important to note that Danazol (17-α-ethinltestosterone), a synthetic androgen that has been used to treat endometriosis, has been revealed to be an independent risk factor for the development of ovarian cancer. A negative correlation between oral contraceptive use and ovarian cancer, regardless of histologic type other than mucinous tumors, was recently shown by a collaboration of various groups worldwide (Cottreau, 2003). These factors may also influence the relative risk of ovarian cancer development.

In addition to an epidemiologic approach, the retrospective pathological analysis of samples from ovarian cancer patients is also useful to confirm the presence of endometriosis associated with ovarian cancers of various histological types. A comprehensive review of 2,807 ovarian cancer patients from 15 independent publications from western countries from the 1970s to 1990s, including 3 articles from Japan, revealed that endometriosis was incidentally found in 14.1% of ovarian cancer patients (39.2%, 21.2%, 3.3% and 3.0% of clear cell, endometrioid, serous and mucinous carcinoma patients, respectively), with a tendency toward a higher incidence of endometriosis in Japanese patients with clear cell carcinoma (Yoshikawa, 2000).

3. Pathogenesis of endometriosis-associated ovarian cancer; the role of iron overload-induced oxidative stress

Endometrial cysts, or so-called chocolate cysts, are well-known lesions in endometriosis that contain fluid with an excess of free iron because of recurring hemorrhage in the cyst. It is interesting to note that Sampson mentioned in his first report of endometriosis-associated cancer that old hemorrhages should be considered additional evidence that meets his criteria (Sampson, 1925). Hemosiderin, heme, or iron deposition in endometriotic lesions have been assumed to trigger oxidative damage and chronic inflammation (Van Langendonckt, 2002a; Van Langendonckt, 2002b; Van Langendonckt, 2004; Toyokuni, 2009). In particular, iron storage in macrophages is significantly increased in patients with endometriosis; and intracellular iron activates the nuclear factor-κB pathway and exaggerates chronic inflammation (Lousse, 2009; Lousse, 2008). As a result, prominent oxidative stress, or an excess of reactive oxygen species, is consistently produced. This process is thought to have a causative role in endometriosis development and progression, leading to carcinogenesis (Murphy, 1998; Ness & Cottreau, 1999; Ngo, 2009). Alternatively, the high concentration of free iron in endometrial cysts may directly provide oxidative stress that induces genomic mutation in epithelial cells (Yamaguchi, 2008), and whether the direct pathway or the indirect pathway involving macrophages has a major role in carcinogenesis remains to be resolved. Iron overload in experimental animals enhances epithelial cell proliferation (Defrere, 2006) and causes malignant tumors with genomic abnormalities (Hu, 2010), which suggests a similar mechanism leading to carcinogenesis in human endometriosis (Fig. 1). However, further studies are awaited to elucidate the precise role of iron-deposition induced oxidative stress in carcinogenesis of endometriosis-associated cancer.

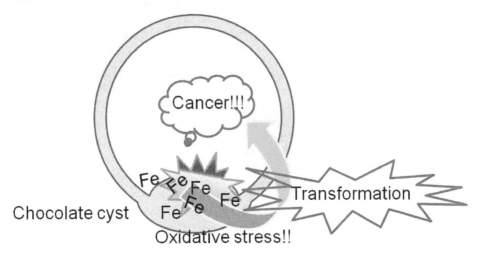

Fig. 1. A proposed mechanism of carcinogenesis in endometriotic (chocolate) cysts

4. Precancerous lesions in endometriosis

Endometriosis itself is generally considered a benign disease; however, endometriosis shares certain features with cancer, including the ability of cells from different lineages (i.e., epithelial cells, stromal cells, and the vasculature) to proliferate in ectopic sites. Thus, earlier studies have focused on the clonal or malignant potential of endometriosis by analyzing the loss of heterozygosity (LOH) at several candidate tumor suppressor gene loci. Positive results, such as the detection of LOH at the p53, p16 or PTEN gene, were observed in the majority of the endometriosis samples ((Jiang, 1996; Jiang, 1998; Sato, 2000), for review of other studies with similar results, see (Prowse, 2005)). Another approach, which assesses the clonality of endometriosis samples by analyzing methylation-related marker genes, also demonstrated the clonal nature of endometriosis (Jimbo, 1997). The findings, together with the LOH analysis, led to the conclusion that endometriosis was a neoplasm that may even have malignant potential. However, recent studies deny the malignant or neoplastic potential of endometriosis, demonstrating that most endometriosis tissues are not monoclonal (Mayr, 2003). Furthermore, neither LOH of tumor suppressor genes, promoter methylation of oncogenes, nor oncogenic mutations of known tumor-related genes was frequently observed in the majority of the cases, further denying the neoplastic theory (Prowse, 2005; Vestergaard AL, 2011). In contrast with these results, a third approach (fluorescent in situ hybridization [FISH]) used to investigate chromosomal aberrations in endometriosis samples revealed a significantly elevated proportion of aneusomic (monosomic > trisomic) cells in endometriosis in multiple groups (Koerner, 2006) (Bischoff, 2002). However, both endometriosis tissue and normal endometrium also contain a certain proportion of aneusomic cells (Koerner, 2006), and telomerase expression, telomere elongation, higher expression of DNA replication markers and lower expression of DNA damage response markers are all observed in endometriosis tissue, but not in normal endometrium (Hapangama, 2008; Hapangama, 2009). Thus, it may be reasonable to conclude that although endometriosis is generally considered non-neoplastic, the relative rates of abnormal cells are higher in endometriosis than in normal endometrium.

In this case, then, which cells are premalignant? Is there a focal area representing the precancerous state of endometriosis that is morphologically distinguishable from other, presumably benign, areas? "Atypical endometriosis" is the term used to describe this state, which has been found in cases of extraovarian and ovarian cancer as atypical epithelium showing hyperchromatism and stratification continuous with the malignant tumor (Brooks&Wheeler, 1977; Lagrenade&Silverberg, 1988). Fukunaga et al. found atypical endometriosis in 61% of endometriosis-associated ovarian cancers, in contrast with 1.7% of benign endometriosis samples (Fukunaga, 1997). Immunohistochemical markers distinguishing atypical endometriosis from benign endometriosis have not been fully established, but staining patterns of Ki67, Bcl-2, and p53 have been reported as useful markers (Nezhat, 2002; Ogawa, 2000). Extraovarian endometriosis may also show atypical changes. Hyperplastic changes, including atypical hyperplasia and malignant changes, were observed in more than half of the adenomyosis cases associated with endometrioid adenocarcinoma arising from the endometrium (Jacques&Lawrence, 1990; Kucera, 2011), and histologically atypical hyperplasia has been reported in some cases of gastrointestinal endometriosis (Yantiss, 2000).

5. Histological characteristics of endometriosis-associated malignancies

Clear cell carcinoma (Fig. 2) and endometrioid adenocarcinoma are well-known histological subtypes in ovarian cancer associated with endometriosis (Fukunaga, 1997; Heaps, 1990; Modesitt, 2002; Ogawa, 2000; Yoshikawa, 2000). Endometrioid adenocarcinoma is the most frequently observed phenotype in western countries (Heaps, 1990; Modesitt, 2002); however, clear cell carcinoma predominates in the Japanese cases (Ogawa, 2000; Yoshikawa, 2000). Veras et al. recently subdivided clear cell carcinoma into 3 groups (cystic, adenofibromatous, and indeterminate clear cell carcinoma) to further reveal the association between endometriosis and cystic clear cell carcinoma subtypes (Veras, 2009). Endometrioid adenocarcinomas arising in endometriotic lesions are often Grade 1 at presentation (Horiuchi, 2003), mostly showing typical morphology with various degrees of squamous differentiation (Heaps, 1990; Staats, 2007), similar to endometrioid adenocarcinoma without endometriosis. Sarcomas are the second and third most frequent endometriosis-associated extraovarian and ovarian tumors, respectively. Adenosarcoma and endometrial stromal sarcoma are the major histological types of sarcomas (Baiocchi, 1990; Heaps, 1990; Slavin, 2000). At least partially, differences in the incidences of tumor types (carcinoma versus sarcoma) depend on the tumor site, and further studies are needed to elucidate this mechanism. Other rare malignant tumors, such as squamous cell carcinoma, malignant mesodermal mixed tumor, and yolk sac tumor, are also reported to develop from endometriosis (Irving, 2011). Although its incidence is very low compared with endometrioid adenocarcinoma or clear cell carcinoma, serous adenocarcinoma has also been associated with endometriosis (Fukunaga, 1997; Modesitt, 2002; Yoshikawa, 2000). Much more rarely, mucinous carcinomas with unusual morphology resembling Mullerian mucinous borderline tumors have also been reported in association with endometriosis (Lee&Nucci, 2003).

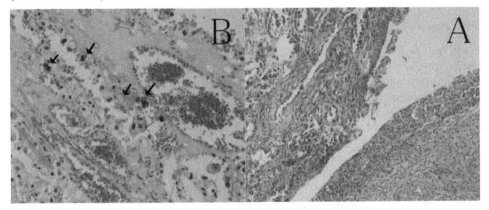

Fig. 2. A. Clear cell carcinoma (left) arising in a endometriotic cyst. B. Hemosiderin deposition (arrows) is observed in the stroma of clear cell carcinoma.

6. Genetic abnormalities and phenotypes of endometriosis-associated ovarian cancer

Genetic mutations specifically associated with ovarian cancer subtypes have been reported (reviewed by (Kurman&Shih, 2011)). Focusing on endometrioid adenocarcinomas, genetic mutations of K-ras, p53, PTEN, beta-catenin, and ATR have been reported (Mizuuchi, 1992; Milner, 1993; Palacios&Gamallo, 1998; Tashiro, 1997; Zighelboim, 2009). Mouse models of endometrioid adenocarcinoma have been reported, either with oncogenic K-ras and conditional PTEN deletion (Dinulescu, 2005) or dysfunction of both the Wnt/beta-catenin and PI3CA/PTEN pathways (Wu, 2007). However, specific genetic alterations of clear cell carcinoma were mostly unknown. Recently, a frequently activated mutation of the PI3CA gene was observed in clear cell carcinoma samples (Kuo, 2009). Most recently, several studies based on novel sequencing technology have elucidated that a significant proportion of clear cell carcinomas harbor a mutation of the ARID1A gene, which encodes the chromatin-remodeling complex protein BAF250A (Jones, 2010; Wiegand, 2010). ARID1A mutation and the consequent loss of BAF250A expression were found not only in clear cell carcinoma samples, but also in endometrioid adenocarcinomas, especially high-grade types

(Wiegand 2010; Wiegand, 2011). Whether ARID1A mutation is an early or late event in endometriosis-associated ovarian cancers related to atypical endometriosis remains to be elucidated. Alterations of other genes, such as p53, p16, and PTEN, have been detected in a low percentage of endometriotic lesions (Martini, 2002; Nezhat, 2008). hMLH, a DNA mismatch repair gene, is another candidate for the malignant transformation of endometriosis (Nyiraneza, 2010 ; Ren F, 2011). hMLH is the causal gene of Lynch syndrome, in which the risk of developing endometrial and ovarian cancers is significantly increased (Schmeler&Lu, 2008). K-ras may also be important because mutated K-ras promotes endometriosis in a mouse model, suggesting that K-ras mutation may be an early event in the carcinogenesis of endometriosis-associated cancers (Cheng, 2011). Finally, a single-nucleotide polymorphism in the intron of ANRIL, a non-coding RNA that regulates p16 expression, has been recently reported to have a strong association with endometriosis (Uno, 2010). The molecular steps from endometriosis development to carcinogenesis remain to be further clarified.

Recent studies have proposed classifying ovarian cancers into two categories: Type I tumors, which rarely harbor the p53 mutation and have an indolent clinical course, and Type II tumors, which feature the p53 mutation and are aggressive (Kurman&Shih, 2010). Within endometriosis-associated ovarian cancers, low-grade endometrioid adenocarcinoma and clear cell carcinomas are considered Type I, while high-grade endometrioid adenocarcinoma is included in the Type II category. However, p53 mutations are detected in both low- and high-grade endometriosis-associated ovarian endometrioid adenocarcinomas (Okuda, 2003), and PI3CA, PPP2R1A, and K-ras mutations are commonly detected in both endometrioid adenocarcinoma and clear cell carcinoma (Campbell, 2004; Jones, 2010 ; Kuo, 2009; McConechy, 2011 ; Mizuuchi, 1992). Recent evidence indicates that ovarian cancers arise from different cell lineages, such as preexisting cystadenomas, ectopic endometrium in endometriotic lesions, and epithelial cells of the Fallopian tubes (Bell, 2005; Kurman&Shih, 2011). Thus, it may be an oversimplification to divide all ovarian cancers into two groups. It may more accurate to categorize endometriosis-associated cancers into the same group, regardless of the histological subtype or tumor grade.

Numerous studies of expression microarray analyses have been published. Cytokines and chemokines, such as interleukin-1 and its downstream factor cyclooxygenase (COX)-2, interleukin-8, TNF-α and its downstream VEGF, TGF- α, and interleukin-6 have been reported to be involved in endometriosis and endometriosis-associated carcinoma (reviewed by (Nezhat, 2008)). An interesting study by Banz et al. revealed that SICA2, CCL14, and TDGF1 were specifically upregulated in both endometriosis samples and endometriosis-associated endometrioid adenocarcinomas, in contrast with serous adenocarcinomas or normal ovarian tissues (Banz, 2010). Another microarray study focusing on endometriosis-associated clear cell carcinoma showed upregulation of hepatocyte nuclear factor (HNF)-1β, versican, and other markers related to oxidative stress (Yamaguchi, 2010). HNF-1β is a transcription factor, involved in the regulation of glucose homeostasis and glycogen accumulation, normally expressed in the liver and other organs, which is assumed to have some role in the pathogenesis of clear cell carcinoma of the ovary (Kobayashi, 2009). Recently, a novel attempt to classify histological subtypes using a small number of biomarkers has been applied to ovarian cancers. A tissue microarray-based analysis selected 21 markers, including CA125, estrogen receptor (ER), insulin-like growth factor 2 (IGF2), Ki-67, p21, p53, progesterone receptor (PGR), and Wilms tumor 1 (WT1), to distinguish histological subtypes; however, only three of the 21 markers could predict outcomes in only high-grade serous carcinoma patients (Koebel, 2008). More recently, however, Kalloger et al. succeeded in reproductively diagnosing five major subtypes of ovarian cancers (high-grade serous, clear cell, endometrioid, mucinous, and low-grade serous) using only nine markers: p16, DKK1 (a Wnt antagonist), HNF-1β, MDM2, PGR, trefoil factor 3 (TFF3), p53, vimentin, and WT1 (Kalloger, 2011). Immunohistochemical analysis of 155 cases by De Lair et al demonstrated that 89% of clear cell carcinoma had HNF-1β positive, ER, PGR, and WT1 negative phenotype (DeLair, 2011).

7. Prognosis of endometriosis-associated ovarian cancer

Clear cell adenocarcinoma is known to be associated with chemoresistancy and a poor prognosis (Itamochi, 2008). However, most reports analyzing the prognosis of endometriosis-associated ovarian carcinomas (including mostly endometrioid adenocarcinoma and few clear cell carcinoma samples) have shown that endometriosis-associated ovarian carcinomas presented at younger ages, in lower grades and stages, and had significantly better overall survival compared with age-matched controls without endometriosis (Erzen, 2001; Kumar, 2011; Melin, 2011 ; Orezzoli, 2008). However, recent studies from various countries indicate that clear cell carcinomas consist of heterogenous tumors with gene alterations, such as HER2 or Met gene amplification (Tan, 2011 ; Yamamoto, 2011; Yamashita, 2011). Therefore, clear cell carcinomas as a subtype are considered to have a worse prognosis than endometrioid adenocarcinomas, especially in Asian cases (Lee, 2011). Recently, the first international symposium of ovarian clear cell carcinoma concluded that although patients with low-stage clear cell carcinoma had a better prognosis than matched controls with high-grade serous carcinoma, high-stage clear cell carcinoma cases had the worst prognosis (Anglesio, 2010). Thus, alternative therapy, such as molecular targeted therapy, should be applied to these aggressive tumors, and a further understanding of the basic biology of the endometriosis-cancer progression, especially the role of oxidative stress, is necessary to prevent carcinogenesis in endometriosis patients (Aris, 2010).

8. Conclusion

We have reviewed the literature on endometriosis-associated ovarian cancer. Further studies are awaited to clarify the exact role of oxidative stress in carcinogenesis.

9. References

Anglesio, M. S., Carey, M. S., Koebel, M., MacKay, H. and Huntsman, D. G. (2010). Clear cell carcinoma of the ovary: A report from the first Ovarian Clear Cell Symposium, June 24th, 2010. *Gynecologic Oncology* 121, 407-415.

Aris, A. (2010). Endometriosis-associated ovarian cancer: A ten-year cohort study of women living in the Estrie Region of Quebec, Canada. *Journal of Ovarian Research* 3, 2.

Baiocchi, G., Kavanagh, J. J. and Wharton, J. T. (1990). Endometrioid Stromal Sarcomas Arising from Ovarian and Extraovarian Endometriosis - Report of 2 Cases and Review of the Literature. *Gynecologic Oncology* 36, 147-151.

Banz, C., Ungethuem, U., Kuban, R.-J., Diedrich, K., Lengyel, E. and Hornung, D. (2010). The molecular signature of endometriosis-associated endometrioid ovarian cancer differs significantly from endometriosis-independent endometrioid ovarian cancer. *Fertility and Sterility* 94, 1212-1217.

Bell, D. A. (2005). Origins and molecular pathology of ovarian cancer. *Modern Pathology* 18, S19-S32.

Bischoff, F. Z., Heard, M. and Simpson, J. L. (2002). Somatic DNA alterations in endometriosis: high frequency of chromosome 17 and p53 loss in late-stage endometriosis. *Journal of Reproductive Immunology* 55, 49-64.

Brinton, L. A., Gridley, G., Persson, I., Baron, J. and Bergqvist, A. (1997). Cancer risk after a hospital discharge diagnosis of endometriosis. *American Journal of Obstetrics and Gynecology* 176, 572-579.

Brooks, J. J. and Wheeler, J. E. (1977). Malignancy Arising in Extra-Gonadal Endometriosis - Case-Report and Summary of World Literature. *Cancer* 40, 3065-3073.

Campbell, I. G., Russell, S. E., Choong, D. Y. H., Montgomery, K. G., Ciavarella, M. L., Hooi, C. S. F., Cristiano, B. E., Pearson, R. B. and Phillips, W. A. (2004). Mutation of the PIK3CA gene in ovarian and breast cancer. *Cancer Research* 64, 7678-7681.

Cheng, C.-w., Licence, D., Cook, E., Luo, F., Arends, M. J., Smith, S. K., Print, C. G. and Charnock-Jones, D. S. (2011). Activation of mutated K-ras in donor endometrial epithelium and stroma promotes lesion growth in an intact immunocompetent murine model of endometriosis. *Journal of Pathology* 224, 261-269.

Cottreau, C. M., Ness, R. B., Modugno, F., Allen, G. O. and Goodman, M. T. (2003). Endometriosis and its treatment with danazol or lupron in relation to ovarian cancer. *Clinical Cancer Research* 9, 5142-5144.

Defrere, S., Van Langendonckt, A., Vaesen, S., Jouret, M., Ramos, R. G., Gonzalez, D. and Donnez, J. (2006). Iron overload enhances epithelial cell proliferation in endometriotic lesions induced in a murine model. *Human Reproduction* 21, 2810-2816.

DeLair, D., Oliva, E., Koebel, M., Macias, A., Gilks, C. B. and Soslow, R. A. (2011). Morphologic Spectrum of Immunohistochemically Characterized Clear Cell Carcinoma of the Ovary: A Study of 155 Cases. *American Journal of Surgical Pathology* 35, 36-44.

Dinulescu, D. M., Ince, T. A., Quade, B. J., Shafer, S. A., Crowley, D. and Jacks, T. (2005). Role of K-ras and Pten in the development of mouse models of endometriosis and endometrioid ovarian cancer. *Nature Medicine* 11, 63-70.

Erzen, M., Rakar, S., Klancar, B. and Syrjanen, K. (2001). Endometriosis-associated ovarian carcinoma (EAOC): An entity distinct from other ovarian carcinomas as suggested by a nested case-control study. *Gynecologic Oncology* 83, 100-108.

Fukunaga, M., Nomura, K., Ishikawa, E. and Ushigome, S. (1997). Ovarian atypical endometriosis: Its close association with malignant epithelial tumours. *Histopathology* 30, 249-255.

Hapangama, D. K., Turner, M. A., Drury, J. A., Quenby, S., Hart, A., Maddick, M., Martin-Ruiz, C. and von Zglinicki, T. (2009). Sustained replication in endometrium of women with endometriosis occurs without evoking a DNA damage response. *Human Reproduction* 24, 687-696.

Hapangama, D. K., Turner, M. A., Drury, J. A., Quenby, S., Saretzki, G., Martin-Ruiz, C. and Von Zglinicki, T. (2008). Endometriosis is associated with aberrant endometrial expression of telomerase and increased telomere length. *Human Reproduction* 23, 1511-1519.

Heaps, J. M., Nieberg, R. K. and Berek, J. S. (1990). Malignant Neoplasms Arising in Endometriosis. *Obstetrics and Gynecology* 75, 1023-1028.

Horiuchi, A., Itoh, K., Shimizu, M., Nakai, I., Yamazaki, T., Kimura, K., Suzuki, A., Shiozawa, I., Ueda, N. and Konishi, I. (2003). Toward understanding the natural history of ovarian carcinoma development: a clinicopathological approach. *Gynecologic Oncology* 88, 309-317.

Hu, Q., Akatsuka, S., Yamashita, Y., Ohara, H., Nagai, H., Okazaki, Y., Takahashi, T. and Toyokuni, S. (2010). Homozygous deletion of CDKN2A/2B is a hallmark of iron-induced high-grade rat mesothelioma. *Laboratory Investigation* 90, 360-373.

Irving, J. A., Clement, P. B. (2011). Diseases of the Peritoneum. *Blaustein's Pathology of the Female Genital Tract. Sixth Edition.*

Itamochi, H., Kigawa, J. and Terakawa, N. (2008). Mechanisms of chemoresistance and poor prognosis in ovarian clear cell carcinoma. *Cancer Science* 99, 653-658.

Jacques, S. M. and Lawrence, W. D. (1990). Endometrial Adenocarcinoma with Variable-Level Myometrial Involvement Limited to Adenomyosis - a Clinicopathological Study of 23 Cases. *Gynecologic Oncology* 37, 401-407.

Jiang, X. X., Hitchcock, A., Bryan, E. J., Watson, R. H., Englefield, P., Thomas, E. J. and Campbell, I. G. (1996). Microsatellite analysis of endometriosis reveals loss of heterozygosity at candidate ovarian tumor suppressor gene loci. *Cancer Research* 56, 3534-3539.

Jiang, X. X., Morland, S. J., Hitchcock, A., Thomas, E. J. and Campbell, I. G. (1998). Allelotyping of endometriosis with adjacent ovarian carcinoma reveals evidence of a common lineage. *Cancer Research* 58, 1707-1712.

Jimbo, H., Hitomi, Y., Yoshikawa, H., Yano, T., Momoeda, M., Sakamoto, A., Tsutsumi, O., Taketani, Y. and Esumi, H. (1997). Evidence for monoclonal expansion of epithelial cells in ovarian endometrial cysts. *American Journal of Pathology* 150, 1173-1178.

Jones, S., Wang, T.-L., Shih, I.-M., Mao, T.-L., Nakayama, K., Roden, R., Glas, R., Slamon, D., Diaz, L. A., Jr., Vogelstein, B., Kinzler, K. W., Velculescu, V. E. and Papadopoulos, N. (2010). Frequent Mutations of Chromatin Remodeling Gene ARID1A in Ovarian Clear Cell Carcinoma. *Science* 330, 228-231.

Kalloger, S. E., Koebel, M., Leung, S., Mehl, E., Gao, D., Marcon, K. M., Chow, C., Clarke, B. A., Huntsman, D. G. and Gilks, C. B. (2011). Calculator for ovarian carcinoma subtype prediction. *Modern Pathology* 24, 512-521.

Kobayashi, H., Sumimoto, K., Moniwa, N., Imai, M., Takakura, K., Kuromaki, T., Morioka, E., Arisawa, K. and Terao, T. (2007). Risk of developing ovarian cancer among women with ovarian endometrioma: a cohort study in Shizuoka, Japan. *International Journal of Gynecological Cancer* 17, 37-43.

Kobayashi, H., Yamada, Y., Kanayama, S., Furukawa, N., Noguchi, T., Haruta, S., Yoshida, S., Sakata, M., Sado, T. and Oi, H. (2009). The Role of Hepatocyte Nuclear Factor-1 beta in the Pathogenesis of Clear Cell Carcinoma of the Ovary. *International Journal of Gynecological Cancer* 19, 471-479.

Koebel, M., Kalloger, S. E., Boyd, N., McKinney, S., Mehl, E., Palmer, C., Leung, S., Bowen, N. J., Ionescu, D. N., Rajput, A., Prentice, L. M., Miller, D., Santos, J., Swenerton, K., Gilks, C. B. and Huntsman, D. (2008). Ovarian Carcinoma Subtypes Are Different Diseases: Implications for Biomarker Studies. *PLoS Medicine* 5, 1749-1760.

Koerner, M., Burckhardt, E. and Mazzucchelli, L. (2006). Higher frequency of chromosomal aberrations in ovarian endometriosis compared to extragonadal endometriosis: a possible link to endometrioid adenocarcinoma. *Modern Pathology* 19, 1615-1623.

Kucera, E., Hejda, V., Dankovcik, R., Valha, P., Dudas, M. and Feyereisl, J. (2011). Malignant changes in adenomyosis in patients with endometrioid adenocarcinoma. *European Journal of Gynaecological Oncology* 32, 182-184.

Kumar, S., Munkarah, A., Arabi, H., Bandyopadhyay, S., Semaan, A., Hayek, K., Garg, G., Morris, R. and Ali-Fehmi, R. (2011). Prognostic analysis of ovarian cancer associated with endometriosis. *American Journal of Obstetrics and Gynecology* 204, 7.

Kuo, K. T., Mao, T. L., Jones, S., Veras, E., Ayhan, A., Wang, T. L., Glas, R., Slamon, D., Velculescu, V. E., Kuman, R. J. and Shih, I. M. (2009). Frequent Activating Mutations of PIK3CA in Ovarian Clear Cell Carcinoma. *American Journal of Pathology* 174, 1597-1601.

Kurman, R. J. and Shih, I.-M. (2010). The Origin and Pathogenesis of Epithelial Ovarian Cancer: A Proposed Unifying Theory. *American Journal of Surgical Pathology* 34, 433-443.

Kurman, R. J. and Shih, I. M. (2011). Molecular pathogenesis and extraovarian origin of epithelial ovarian cancer-Shifting the paradigm. *Human Pathology* 42, 918-931.

Lagrenade, A. and Silverberg, S. G. (1988). Ovarian-Tumors Associated with Atypical Endometriosis. *Human Pathology* 19, 1080-1084.

Lee, K. R. and Nucci, M. R. (2003). Ovarian mucinous and mixed epithelial carcinomas of mullerian (endocervical-like) type: A clinicopathologic analysis of four cases of an uncommon variant associated with endometriosis. *International Journal of Gynecological Pathology* 22, 42-51.

Lee, Y.-Y., Kim, T.-J., Kim, M.-J., Kim, H.-J., Song, T., Kim, M. K., Choi, C. H., Lee, J.-W., Bae, D.-S. and Kim, B.-G. (2011). Prognosis of ovarian clear cell carcinoma compared to other histological subtypes: A meta-analysis. *Gynecologic Oncology* 122, 541-547.

Lousse, J.-C., Defrere, S., Van Langendonckt, A., Gras, J., Gonzalez-Ramos, R., Colette, S. and Donnez, J. (2009). Iron storage is significantly increased in peritoneal macrophages of endometriosis patients and correlates with iron overload in peritoneal fluid. *Fertility and Sterility* 91, 1668-1675.

Lousse, J.-C., Van Langendonckt, A., Gonzalez-Ramos, R., Defrere, S., Renkin, E. and Donnez, J. (2008). Increased activation of nuclear factor-kappa B (NF-kappa B) in isolated peritoneal macrophages of patients with, endometriosis. *Fertility and Sterility* 90, 217-220.

Martini, M., Ciccarone, M., Garganese, G., Maggiore, C., Evangelista, A., Rahimi, S., Zannoni, G., Vittori, G. and Larocca, L. M. (2002). Possible involvement of hMLH1, p16(INK4a) and PTEN in the malignant transformation of endometriosis. *International Journal of Cancer* 102, 398-406.

Mayr, D., Amann, G., Siefert, C., Diebold, J. and Anderegg, B. (2003). Does endometriosis really have premalignant potential? A clonal analysis of laser-microdissected tissue. *Faseb Journal* 17, 693-+.

McConechy, M. K., Anglesio, M. S., Kalloger, S. E., Yang, W., Senz, J., Chow, C., Heravi-Moussavi, A., Morin, G. B., Mes-Masson, A.-M., Carey, M. S., McAlpine, J. N., Kwon, J. S., Prentice, L. M., Boyd, N., Shah, S. P., Gilks, C. B. and Huntsman, D. G. (2011). Subtype-specific mutation of PPP2R1A in endometrial and ovarian carcinomas. *Journal of Pathology* 223, 567-573.

Melin, A., Lundholm, C., Malki, N., Swahn, M. L., Sparen, P. and Bergqvist, A. (2011). Endometriosis as a prognostic factor for cancer survival. *International Journal of Cancer* 129, 948-955.

Milner, B. J., Allan, L. A., Eccles, D. M., Kitchener, H. C., Leonard, R. C. F., Kelly, K. F., Parkin, D. E. and Haites, N. E. (1993). P53 Mutation Is a Common Genetic Event in Ovarian-Carcinoma. *Cancer Research* 53, 2128-2132.

Mizuuchi, H., Nasim, S., Kudo, R., Silverberg, S. G., Greenhouse, S. and Garrett, C. T. (1992). Clinical Implications of K-Ras Mutations in Malignant Epithelial Tumors of the Endometrium. *Cancer Research* 52, 2777-2781.

Modesitt, S. C., Tortoler-Luna, G., Robinson, J. B., Gershenson, D. M. and Wolf, J. K. (2002). Ovarian and extraovarian endometriosis-associated cancer. *Obstetrics and Gynecology* 100, 788-795.

Murphy, A. A., Santanam, N. and Parthasarathy, S. (1998). Endometriosis: A disease of oxidative stress? *Seminars in Reproductive Endocrinology* 16, 263-273.

Nagle, C. M., Olsen, C. M., Webb, P. M., Jordan, S. J., Whiteman, D. C. and Green, A. C. (2008). Endometrioid and clear cell ovarian cancers - A comparative analysis of risk factors. *European Journal of Cancer* 44, 2477-2484.

Ness, R. B. and Cottreau, C. (1999). Possible role of ovarian epithelial inflammation in ovarian cancer. *Journal of the National Cancer Institute* 91, 1459-1467.

Ness, R. B., Grisso, J. A., Cottreau, C., Klapper, J., Vergona, R., Wheeler, J. E., Morgan, M. and Schlesselman, J. J. (2000). Factors related to inflammation of the ovarian epithelium and risk of ovarian cancer. *Epidemiology* 11, 111-117.

Nezhat, F., Cohen, C., Rahaman, J., Gretz, H., Cole, P. and Kalir, T. (2002). Comparative immunohistochemical studies of bcl-2 and p53 proteins in benign and malignant ovarian endometriotic cysts. *Cancer* 94, 2935-2940.

Nezhat, F., Datta, M. S., Hanson, V., Pejovic, T., Nezhat, C. and Nezhat, C. (2008). The relationship of endometriosis and ovarian malignancy: a review. *Fertility and Sterility* 90, 1559-1570.

Ngo, C., Chereau, C., Nicco, C., Weill, B., Chapron, C. and Batteux, F. (2009). Reactive Oxygen Species Controls Endometriosis Progression. *American Journal of Pathology* 175, 225-234.

Nyiraneza, C., Marbaix, E., Smets, M., Galant, C., Sempoux, C. and Dahan, K. (2010). High risk for neoplastic transformation of endometriosis in a carrier of lynch syndrome. *Familial Cancer* 9, 383-387.

Ogawa, S., Kaku, T., Amada, S., Kobayashi, H., Hirakawa, T., Ariyoshi, K., Kamura, T. and Nakano, H. (2000). Ovarian endometriosis associated with ovarian carcinoma: A clinicopathological and immunohistochemical study. *Gynecologic Oncology* 77, 298-304.

Okuda, T., Otsuka, J., Sekizawa, A., Saito, H., Makino, R., Kushima, M., Farina, A., Kuwano, Y. and Okai, T. (2003). p53 mutations and overexpression affect prognosis of ovarian endometrioid cancer but not clear cell cancer. *Gynecologic Oncology* 88, 318-325.

Orezzoli, J. P., Russell, A. H., Oliva, E., Del Carmen, M. G., Eichhorn, J. and Fuller, A. F. (2008). Prognostic implication of endometriosis in clear cell carcinoma of the ovary. *Gynecologic Oncology* 110, 336-344.

Palacios, J. and Gamallo, C. (1998). Mutations in the beta-catenin gene (CTNNB1) in endometrioid ovarian carcinomas. *Cancer Research* 58, 1344-1347.

Postoloff, A. V. and Rodenberg, T. A. (1955). Malignant Transition in Ovarian Endometriosis. *American Journal of Obstetrics and Gynecology* 69, 83-86.

Prowse, A. H., Fakis, G., Manek, S., Churchman, M., Edwards, S., Rowan, A., Koninckx, P., Kennedy, S. and Tomlinson, I. P. M. (2005). Allelic loss studies do not provide evidence for the "endometriosis-as-tumor" theory. *Fertility and Sterility* 83, 1134-1143.

Ren F, W. D., Jiang Y, Ren F (2011). Epigenetic inactivation of hMLH1 in the malignant transformation of ovarian endometriosis. *Archives of Gynecology and Obstetrics*. [Epub ahead of print].

Sampson, J. A. (1925). Endometrial carcinoma of the ovary, arising in endometrial tissue in that organ. *Archives of Surgery* 10, 1-72.

Sato, N., Tsunoda, H., Nishida, M., Morishita, Y., Takimoto, Y., Kubo, T. and Noguchi, M. (2000). Loss of heterozygosity on 10q23.3 and mutation of the tumor suppressor gene PTEN in benign endometrial cyst of the ovary: Possible sequence progression from benign endometrial cyst to endometrioid carcinoma and clear cell carcinoma of the ovary. *Cancer Research* 60, 7052-7056.

Schmeler, K. M. and Lu, K. H. (2008). Gynecologic cancers associated with Lynch syndrome/HNPCC. *Clinical & Translational Oncology* 10, 313-317.

Scott, R. B. (1953). Malignant Changes in Endometriosis. *Obstetrics and Gynecology* 2, 283-289.

Slavin, R. E., Krum, R. and Van Dinh, T. (2000). Endometriosis-associated intestinal tumors: A clinical and pathological study of 6 cases with a review of the literature. *Human Pathology* 31, 456-463.

Staats, P. N., Clement, P. B. and Young, R. H. (2007). Primary endometrioid adenocarcinoma of the vagina - A clinicopathologic study of 18 cases. *American Journal of Surgical Pathology* 31, 1490-1501.

Tan, D. S. P., Iravani, M., McCluggage, W. G., Lambros, M. B. K., Milanezi, F., Mackay, A., Gourley, C., Geyer, F. C., Vatcheva, R., Millar, J., Thomas, K., Natrajan, R., Savage, K., Fenwick, K., Williams, A., Jameson, C., El-Bahrawy, M., Gore, M. E., Gabra, H., Kaye, S. B., Ashworth, A. and Reis-Filho, J. S. (2011). Genomic Analysis Reveals the Molecular Heterogeneity of Ovarian Clear Cell Carcinomas. *Clinical Cancer Research* 17, 1521-1534.

Tashiro, H., Blazes, M. S., Wu, R., Cho, K. R., Bose, S., Wang, S. I., Li, J., Parsons, R. and Ellenson, L. H. (1997). Mutations in PTEN are frequent in endometrial carcinoma but rare in other common gynecological malignancies. *Cancer Research* 57, 3935-3940.

Toyokuni, S. (2009). Role of iron in carcinogenesis: Cancer as a ferrotoxic disease. *Cancer Science* 100, 9-16.

Uno, S., Zembutsu, H., Hirasawa, A., Takahashi, A., Kubo, M., Akahane, T., Aoki, D., Kamatani, N., Hirata, K. and Nakamura, Y. (2010). A genome-wide association study identifies genetic variants in the CDKN2BAS locus associated with endometriosis in Japanese. *Nature Genetics* 42, 707-U788.

Van Langendonckt, A., Casanas-Roux, F., Dolmans, M.-M. and Donnez, J. (2002a). Potential involvement of hemoglobin and heme in the pathogenesis of peritoneal endometriosis. *Fertility and Sterility* 77, 561-570.

Van Langendonckt, A., Casanas-Roux, F. and Donnez, J. (2002b). Iron overload in the peritoneal cavity of women with pelvic endometriosis. *Fertility and Sterility* 78, 712-718.

Van Langendonckt, A., Casanas-Roux, F., Eggermont, J. and Donnez, J. (2004). Characterization of iron deposition in endometriotic lesions induced in the nude mouse model. *Human Reproduction* 19, 1265-1271.

Veras, E., Mao, T.-L., Ayhan, A., Ueda, S., Lai, H., Hayran, M., Shih, I.-M. and Kurman, R. J. (2009). Cystic and Adenofibromatous Clear Cell Carcinomas of the Ovary Distinctive Tumors That Differ in Their Pathogenesis and Behavior: A Clinicopothologic Analysis of 122 Cases. *American Journal of Surgical Pathology* 33, 844-853.

Vestergaard AL, T. K., Knudsen UB, Munk T, Rosbach H, Poulsen JB, Guldberg P, Martensen PM. (2011). Oncogenic events associated with endometrial and ovarian cancers are rare in endometriosis. *Molecular Human Reproduction* [Epub ahead of print].

Wiegand, K. C., Lee, A. F., Al-Agha, O. M., Chow, C., Kalloger, S. E., Scott, D. W., Steidl, C., Wiseman, S. M., Gascoyne, R. D., Gilks, B. and Huntsman, D. G. (2011). Loss of BAF250a (ARID1A) is frequent in high-grade endometrial carcinomas. *Journal of Pathology* 224, 328-333.

Wiegand, K. C., Shah, S. P., Al-Agha, O. M., Zhao, Y., Tse, K., Zeng, T., Senz, J., McConechy, M. K., Anglesio, M. S., Kalloger, S. E., Yang, W., Heravi-Moussavi, A., Giuliany, R., Chow, C., Fee, J., Zayed, A., Prentice, L., Melnyk, N., Turashvili, G., Delaney, A. D., Madore, J., Yip, S., McPherson, A. W., Ha, G., Bell, L., Fereday, S., Tam, A., Galletta, L., Tonin, P. N., Provencher, D., Miller, D., Jones, S. J. M., Moore, R. A., Morin, G. B., Oloumi, A., Boyd, N., Aparicio, S. A., Shih, I.-M., Mes-Masson, A.-M., Bowtell, D. D., Hirst, M., Gilks, B., Marra, M. A. and Huntsman, D. G. (2010). ARID1A Mutations in Endometriosis-Associated Ovarian Carcinomas. *New England Journal of Medicine* 363, 1532-1543.

Wu, R., Hendrix-Lucas, N., Kuick, R., Zhai, Y., Schwartz, D. R., Akyol, A., Hanash, S., Misek, D. E., Katabuchi, H., Williams, B. O., Fearon, E. R. and Cho, K. R. (2007). Mouse model of human ovarian endometrioid adenocarcinoma based on somatic defects in the Wnt/beta-catenin and PI3K/Pten signaling pathways. *Cancer Cell* 11, 321-333.

Yamaguchi, K., Mandai, M., Oura, T., Matsumura, N., Hamanishi, J., Baba, T., Matsui, S., Murphy, S. K. and Konishi, I. (2010). Identification of an ovarian clear cell carcinoma gene signature that reflects inherent disease biology and the carcinogenic processes. *Oncogene* 29, 1741-1752.

Yamaguchi, K., Mandai, M., Toyokuni, S., Hamanishi, J., Higuchi, T., Takakura, K. and Fujii, S. (2008). Contents of endometriotic cysts, especially the high concentration of free iron, are a possible cause of carcinogenesis in the cysts through the iron-induced persistent oxidative stress. *Clinical Cancer Research* 14, 32-40.

Yamamoto, S., Tsuda, H., Miyai, K., Takano, M., Tamai, S. and Matsubara, O. (2011). Gene amplification and protein overexpression of MET are common events in ovarian clear-cell adenocarcinoma: their roles in tumor progression and prognostication of the patient. *Modern Pathology* 24, 1146-1155.

Yamashita, Y., Yatabe, Y., Akatsuka, S., Kajiyama, H., Kikkawa, F. ,Takahashi, T., and Toyokuni, S. (2011) MET amplification is a molecular hallmark in endometriosis-associated ovarian clear cell carcinoma and correlates with worse prognosis. *European Journal of Cancer* 47, S529-S529

Yantiss, R. K., Clement, P. B. and Young, R. H. (2000). Neoplastic and pre-neoplastic changes in gastrointestinal endometriosis - A study of 17 cases. *American Journal of Surgical Pathology* 24, 513-524.

Yoshikawa, H., Jimbo, H., Okada, S., Matsumoto, K., Onda, T., Yasugi, T. and Taketani, Y. (2000). Prevalence of endometriosis in ovarian cancer. *Gynecologic and Obstetric Investigation* 50, 11-15.

Zighelboim, I., Schmidt, A. P., Gao, F., Thaker, P. H., Powell, M. A., Rader, J. S., Gibb, R. K., Mutch, D. G. and Goodfellow, P. J. (2009). ATR Mutation in Endometrioid Endometrial Cancer Is Associated With Poor Clinical Outcomes. *Journal of Clinical Oncology* 27, 3091-3096.

4

Alteration in Endometrial Remodeling: A Cause for Implantation Failure in Endometriosis?

Saikat K. Jana, Priyanka Banerjee, Shyam Thangaraju,
Baidyanath Chakravarty and Koel Chaudhury
Indian Institute of Technology, Kharagpur,
India

1. Introduction

1.1 Implantation failure in endometriosis

The process of implantation is an interactive cascade of events between the embryo and the endometrium. It is a dynamic process consisting of three distinct phases. They are (i) apposition of embryo (ii) attachment with the epithelial lining of the endometrium and (iii) invasion into the endometrial stroma gaining access to the maternal circulatory system. Embryo implantation failure may occur due to embryonic defect or unsupportive endometrium. Advances in Assisted Reproductive Technology (ART) have made it possible to obtain good quality embryos; however, successful implantation remains the bottleneck for a successful pregnancy. The endometrium remodels before attaining a state of receptivity. Endometrium remains receptive during a limited period, when it is favourable for blastocyst attachment and implantation. In women, there is clinical evidence of a brief period of optimal uterine receptivity which allows for blastocyst implantation. This period, called the implantation window, is related to changes in the endometrial epithelial morphology. Inappropriate morphological development leads to unreceptive endometrium that causes defective endometrial /embryonic cross talk. This is generally agreed to be one of the main reasons for implantation failure. Endometriosis, characterized by benign growth of endometrial tissue outside the uterus, affects approximately 20%–48% of women during their reproductive years. The occurrence of aberrant hormonal, immunological, genetic and pathophysiological events associated with endometriosis is attributed to the heterogeneous etiology of the disease. The symptoms of endometriosis do not depend on the severity or stage of the disease. Women with even mildest degree of endometriosis can have a 3 – 4 fold reduction in their annual birth rate compared to normal non-endometriotic women.

Presence of endometriosis alters the characteristic of the endometrium. It also affects the expression of various factors and markers of receptivity during implantation window. All these result in dysfunctional endometrium. This can be a cause of higher implantation failure rates and lower pregnancy rates in endometriotic women due to failure of embryo implantation. However, alterations in endometrial remodeling in endometriosis resulting in impairment of the endometrial receptivity is still poorly understood. An understanding of endometrial receptivity in women with endometriosis is, therefore, crucial in understanding the fundamental causes of implantation failure which in turn, may have significant implications on fertility potential of these women.

2. Matrix turnover and angiogenesis during implantation

2.1 Matrix turnover in endometrium and implantation

The unique characteristic of the endometrial tissue is that it undergoes cyclic degeneration and regeneration in each menstrual cycle. The endometrium consists of a layer of columnar epithelium bedded on a layer of connective tissue. The extracellular matrix (ECM), which forms a component of the connective tissue, provides the scaffolding for the anchorage of the cells within the tissue (McIntush and Smith 1998) and presents a locale for cellular migration, division and differentiation (Birkedal-Hansen et al., 1993). The extensive remodeling of the connective tissue of the endometrium requires both the degradation and reformation of the ECM which is accomplished by highly regulated turnover of the ECM (Hulboy et al., 1997). This destruction of the ECM occurs by the action of a class of proteolytic enzyme identified as matrix metalloproteinases (MMP). MMPs and the tissue inhibitors of metalloproteinases (TIMP) regulate a number of aspects of reproductive physiology like dynamic remodeling of the ovary and endometrium throughout each menstrual cycle, implantation, embryonic development and parturition. There exists equilibrium between the MMPs and TIMPs action for controlling this turnover of the ECM. Any circumstances that may bring about interruption of this delicate balance leads to a number of pathological complexities related to pregnancy and infertility like luteinized unruptured follicle syndrome, ovarian cysts, endometriosis, uterine fibroids, inappropriate implantation resulting in tubal pregnancy or spontaneous abortion, premature rupture of fetal membranes, or carcinoma of the ovary or uterus (Curry and Osteen 2003).

Several studies have reported the diverse pattern of MMPs expression in the endometrium throughout the menstrual cycle. Since breakdown of the endometrial lining occurs during menstruation, several MMPs are reported to be highly expressed during this phase. However, their expression gradually falls off during rest of the cycle. Nevertheless various MMPs are observed to express at various phases of the cycling endometrium. Expression of MMP-2 remains consistent throughout the whole cycle along with TIMP-1 and TIMP-2. Endometrial MMP-9 expression shows a cyclical change in its distribution between glandular and stromal cells. It expresses in the endometrium throughout the cycle, however, its expression increases during midsecretory phase particularly in the glandular cells (Hulboy et al., 1997). Although the association of MMP-2 and -9 and their endogenous inhibitors in pathogenesis of infertile condition like endometriosis is well established (Salata et al., 2008), knowledge regarding their involvement in endometrial remodelling during implantation window in endometriotic women is limited.

2.2 Angiogenesis

Endometrial remodeling involves proliferation of its functional layer upon estrogen enhancement (Groothuis et al., 2007) and differentiation by the influence of progesterone from the luteinized follicles (Okada et al., 1999). This is followed by the degeneration of this superficial layer and again reconstruction of the new one. These constant cyclic changes of the endometrium are associated with angiogenesis and neovascularisation (Perrot-Applanat et al., 2000). Vascular endothelial growth factor (VEGF) is a prime angiogenic stimulus for vascular permeability based on its capability to bring on vascular leakage (Ferrara and Davis-Smyth 1997, Ferrara et al., 2003). VEGF regulated angiogenesis and neovasculogenesis of the endometrial tissue is elemental for the growth and differentiation of the endometrium for implantation and placentation (Giudice 1996, Perrot-Applanat 2000). Due to its control over the human reproductive cycle, VEGF is present in the stromal and glandular epithelium of the human endometrium throughout all phases of the menstrual cycle (Torry and Torry 1997, Smith 1998, Shifren et al., 1996, Charnock-Jones 1993, Popovici 1999, Lockwood 2002). However there exists a strong debate regarding its expression and angiogenesis. VEGF expression increased in the late secretory phase and heightened during menses (Torry and Torry 1997, Charnock-Jones 1993, Popovici 1999, Lockwood 2002, Bausero 1998). There is a marked increase even in the vascular network of the endometrium during the secretory phase over the proliferative phase (Ota 1998). But Nayak and Brenner reported that during proliferative phase there is a noted increase in the VEGF expression in stroma which shifts to glandular epithelium during the secretory phase (Nayak and Brenner 2002). However, contradictory report exist indicating that a gradual decline in angiogenesis occurs at the end of the cycle which rapidly increases with the start of a new cycle and reaching a maximum height during the mid cycle (Au and Rogers 1993). Other investigators have suggested that VEGF expression remains inconsistent (Sugino et al., 2002) or there is no change in the vascularity throughout the endometrial cycle (Rogers and Au 1993).

2.3 Regulation of matrix remodeling

It is suggested that inappropriate regulation of sex steroids may lead to defect in implantation. The role of estradiol in embryo implantation is a subject of controversy and its association with pregnancy outcome in IVF cycle is an area of research for many years (Kyrou et al 2009). Several studies have shown that midluteal decline of serum estradiol do not affect the endometrial development, embryo implantation and IVF outcome (Friedler et al., 2005; Narvekar et al., 2010; Hung et al., 2000). This may be due to the fact that during follicular phase, estradiol induces growth of follicles, preparation of endometrium and production of specific proteins, growth factors and receptors of estrogen and progesterone. Additionally, adverse effect of high estradiol level on endometrial receptivity is still under debate (Kyrou et al., 2009). A number of investigators found no effect of high estradiol levels on the treatment outcome of IVF/ICSI cycle (Sharara and McClamrock 1999, Kosmas et al., 2004). Some studies have, however, suggested that elevated levels of estradiol may be responsible for impaired endometrial receptivity (Simon et al., 1995; Valbuena et al., 2001; Kyrou et al., 2009). After ovulation, progesterone is the main contributory sex hormone executing the transformation of the endometrium during the secretory phase.

It is evidenced that expression of cyclooxygenase-2 (COX-2), a molecule associated with angiogenesis and cell differentiation, promotes the release of MMP-2 (Xiong et al., 2005) and -9 (Itatsu et al., 2009), and angiogenic factor VEGF (Wang et al. (2010). COX-2, on the other hand, is regulated by female sexual hormone estradiol and progesterone (Li et al., 2007). Since the process of angiogenesis during endometrial remodelling shares similarities with the process of angiogenesis during metastasis in cancer, estradiol may also be involved in the up-regulation of the gene expression of COX-2 and MMPs during embryo implantation. Involvement of COX-2 gene in embryo implantation is a subject of interest among the researchers working on endometrial receptivity, and is suggested to play an important regulatory role in successful implantation. However, little is known about its role in endometrial receptivity in women with endometriosis.

2.4 Endometrial receptivity markers

Inadequate uterine receptivity and poor embryo formation are two major factors responsible for implantation failure (Simon et al., 1998; Ledee-Bataille et al., 2002). Nowadays, using

ART procedure, clinicians can improve embryo formation considerably; however, no therapies are available to make the endometrium more receptive. Expression of various implantation markers and proteins lead to remodeling of the endometrial matrix thereby transforming the endometrium towards a receptive milieu. Several molecular repertoires expressed during the implantation window are considered to be useful markers of implantation. Expression of various markers including pinopodes $\alpha_v\beta_3$ integrin, LIF, L-selectin ligand and Mucin-1 throughout the different stages of implantation are considered to be responsible for endometrial receptivity.

2.4.1 Pinopodes

Pinopodes, also known as uterodomes, are large cytoplasmic protrusions from the endometrial epithelial surface and are several micrometers wide. These are specialized cell structures that are involved in adhesion and penetration of the blastocyst into the stroma. These structures project into the uterine lumen and are above the microvilli level. Their expression is limited to a maximum period of 2 days during the menstrual cycle corresponding to the presumed window of implantation (Stavreus-Evers et al., 2001). Endometrial pinopodes development is associated with the mid-luteal phase increased expression of leukaemia inhibitory factor (LIF) and its receptor (Aghajanova et al., 2003), progesterone (Stavreus-Evers et al., 2001) and integrin $\alpha_v\beta_3$ (Lessey et al., 1992). Advocated as a marker of uterine receptivity, their expression, has been investigated solely by means of scanning electron microscopy (SEM) (Develioglu et al., 2000).

2.4.2 Integrins

Integrins are surface ligands, usually glycoproteins, belonging to the class of cell adhesion molecules (CAM). An integrin molecule consists of two different, non-covalently linked α and β subunits that are paired to form various heterodimers with distinct function (Hynes, 2002). At least 20 types of integrin heterodimer have been defined, which form from 14α and 9β subunits (Lindhard 2002). Integrins are unusual cell surface receptors in that they bind with low affinity and are present in large numbers, allowing for ligand motility without loss of attachment. Endometrial epithelial cells constitutively express certain integrins, whereas others are cycle dependent (Lessey 1992). $\alpha_v\beta_3$, an example of the latter is present on the apical surface of both luminal endometrial cells and human embryos. 41 different aberrant expressions of this integrin are reported in women with endometriosis (Lessey et al., 1994).

2.4.3 LIF

LIF is a member of the IL-6 family and is secreted by the endometrial epithelium, CD16–CD56 natural killer cells and type 2 T-helper cells. Animal and human studies indicate that LIF plays an important role in implantation and for pregnancy to occur (Lass et al., 2001). LIF protein can be detected by immunohistochemistry in the luminal, glandular and stromal epithelium. There is very little LIF expression in proliferative endometrium, but levels increase during the secretory phase, reaching a maximum between days 19 and 25, which coincides with the implantation window (Charnock-Jones 1994).

2.4.4 Mucins

Mucins are high molecular weight (MW) glycoproteins, which contain at least 50% of carbohydrate O-linked to a threonine/serine rich peptide core (Gendler et al., 1990). Among the 14 cloned human mucins, only Mucin-1 (MUC1) and to a lesser extent MUC6 have been found in the human endometrium (Gipson et al., 1997). Cell–cell and cell–matrix adhesion are inhibited in direct correlation to the length of the MUC-1 ectodomain (Hilkens et al., 1992; Wesseling et al., 1996).

2.4.5 L-Selectin ligand

Selectins are glycoproteins which also belong to the CAM family. The expression of selectin oligosaccharide-based ligands, such as MECA-79 or HECA-452, is up-regulated during the window of implantation (Genbacev et al., 2003). MECA-79 is immunolocalized in the luminal and glandular endometrial epithelium throughout the menstrual cycle, although the staining considerably intensifies during the mid-secretory phase. The physiological importance of the interaction between L-selectin and its oligosaccharide ligands has been investigated in the human endometrium (Genbacev et al., 2003).

Though several studies investigating endometrial receptivity during implantation window are documented, the mechanism responsible for implantation failure in endometriosis is still poorly understood. Expression of various cell adhesion molecules and pinopodes in women with endometriosis is explored in the present study. Since, COX-2 is reported to be physiologically involved in the process of angiogenesis (Matsumoto et al., 2002), and in view of the fact that angiogenesis is essential for endometrial remodeling, we were motivated to assess the expression of various angiogenic factors including VEGFR, MMP-2,-9 and their tissue inhibitors in women with endometriosis during the implantation window. Additionally, expression of COX-2 was studied to assess their associated regulatory role in the process of endometrial remodeling during implantation window.

2.5 Material and method

2.5.1 Subject selection

30 women with endometriosis and 20 without the disease were included in the study. Presence/absence of endometriosis was confirmed by diagnostic laparoscopy. It was ensured that these women had not received any kind of medical or hormonal treatment during the past three months. Women with history of chocolate cyst removal, previous history of any surgery, with other possible causes of pain or pelvic pathology including pelvic tuberculosis were excluded.

2.5.2 Sample collection

Blood samples collected from patients were allowed to clot and the serum separated by centrifugation at 3,000 rpm for 5 min at 4°C. Serum samples were stored at -20°C until further use. Endometrial biopsy was performed on the 7th day after confirmation of ovulation. The collected tissue was washed in phosphate buffer saline (PBS) and divided into three parts: one part was used for stromal and epithelial cells isolation for flow cytometric analysis of different molecular repertoires of the endometrium, the other part was fixed for immunohistochemistry (IHC) and scanning electron microscopy of these receptivity markers. From the third part, RNA was isolated immediately.

2.5.3 Isolation of cells and flow cytometric analysis

Endometrial tissue was first digested in 2% collagenase-1 (Invitrogen, Grand Island, NY, USA) in DMEM (Himedia, Mumbai, India) for 1.5 to 2 hrs at 37°C and then centrifuged to isolate the stromal cells. Undigested glands were then treated with 0.25% trypsin-0.02% EDTA (Himedia, Mumbai, India) for 4–8min, washed with 10% FBS-DMEM. Single epithelial cells were isolated by centrifugation, as described previously. Isolated cells were washed, RBC lysed using RBC lysis solution and fixed in 2% paraformaldehyde (20 min at RT). Single cell suspension thus obtained was divided into five parts; four parts were stained with mouse anti-human $\alpha_v\beta_3$ integrin, LIF (R&D Systems, Minneapolis, MN, USA), Muc-1 (Abcam, Cambridge, UK) and rat anti-human MECA-79 monoclonal antibody (Santa Cruz 1 Biotechnology, Inc., Santa Cruz, California, USA) according to instructions provided by the manufacturer in the manual. The fifth part remained unstained. Excess antibodies were washed out and the cells again incubated with fluorescein conjugated secondary goat anti-mouse and anti-rat IgG (R&D Systems, Minneapolis, MN, USA). After washing excess antibodies, the stained cells were analyzed using flow cytometer (BD FACS Calibur™, BD Biosciences, San Jose, CA, USA).

2.5.4 Immunohistochemistry

3-5 μm thick sections obtained from formaldehyde fixed, paraffin-embedded tissue were dehydrated in graded ethanol. After antigen retrieval, slides were blocked using 3% BSA in PBS and incubated with mouse anti-human $\alpha v\beta 3$ integrin (R&D Systems, Minneapolis, MN, USA), Muc-1 (Abcam, Cambridge, UK), LIF and rat anti-human MECA-79 monoclonal antibody (Santa Cruz biotechnology, INC., Santa Cruz, California, USA). Excess primary antibody was washed with PBS and the sections were again incubated with anti-mouse and anti-rat biotinylated secondary antibody (Santa Cruz biotechnology, INC., Santa Cruz, California, USA) according to the manufacturer's protocol, before incubation with avidin biotinylated horseradish peroxidase (Santa Cruz biotechnology, INC., Santa Cruz, California, USA). Labeled cells were visualized with Diaminobenzidine (DAB) and sections counterstained with hematoxylin. Next, the slides were dehydrated using series of alcohol gradient and mounted using distrene, tricresyl phosphate (DPX) and xylene. The slides were then examined under bright field microscope (Carl Zeiss, Jena, Germany).

2.5.5 Scanning electron microscopy

Formaldehyde-fixed tissues were washed in PBS and dehydrated in a series of alcohol gradient (50%, 70%, 90%, 95%, 100%), each for 10 mins, dipped in HMDS (1,1,1,3,3,3-hexamethyl disilazane; SRL, Bombay, India) and air dried. Dried tissues were then mounted and coated with gold and the luminal endometrial surface thoroughly examined under SEM (Jeol JSM-5800 Scanning Microscope, Tokyo, Japan). Pinopode formation was also evaluated semi-quantitatively depending on their stage of development on the surface of the endometrium, and scored as (i) well-developed (ii) poorly developed and (iii) absent and on their abundance and scored as (i) abundant (ii) moderate (iii) few.

2.5.6 Real-time PCR

Levels of COX-2, MMP-2, -9, TIMP-1 and -2 gene expression were analyzed by real time PCR (RT-PCR), which was performed with ABI Prism 7000 Sequence Detection System (Applied Biosystems Inc., Carlsbad, California, USA) using syber green master mix (Applied Biosystems Inc., Carlsbad, California, USA). RT-PCR primers were designed using sequence data. Total RNA was isolated from tissue by RNA isolation kit (Trizol Reagent, Invitrogen, Carlsbad, California, USA) and 10 µl of total RNA isolated was subjected to reverse transcription for cDNA synthesis with High-Capacity cDNA Reverse Transcription Kits (Applied Biosystems, Carlsbad, California, USA), according to the manufacturer's instructions. After synthesis, 5 µl of cDNA was used for the RT-PCR mixed with syber green. At the end of each reaction, Cycle threshold (Ct) was manually set at the level that reflected the best kinetic PCR parameters, and melting curves were acquired and analyzed. Relative quantification was used to measure gene expression by relating the PCR signal.

2.5.7 Western blotting

The endometrial tissue was homogenized in tissue lysis buffer. The tissue lysate was then centrifuged at 15,000 g for 15 min and the protein concentration of the homogenates was determined by the GeNei™ Protein Estimation Kits (Bangalore Genei, India). 30 µg of homogenate protein were separated by SDS-polyacrylamide gel electrophoresis (SDS- PAGE). The separated proteins were electroblotted onto a Hybond PVDF membrane (GE Healthcare) at 30 volt for 13 hrs. After blocking the non-specific binding sites with non-fat dry milk in TBST buffer for 1 hr at room temperature, the blots were incubated overnight at 4°C with rabbit polyclonal antibody against COX-2, mouse monoclonal antibody against MMP-2,-9, TIMP-1 and -2 (Santa Cruz Biotechnology Inc, Santa Cruz, CA, USA), rabbit polyclonal antibody against VEGF, VEGFR1+VEGFR2 (Abcam, Cambridge, UK). The blots were then washed three times with TBST buffer, incubated for 1 hr at room temperature with horseradish peroxidase-linked goat anti-rabbit immunoglobulin G (IgG) and goat anti-mouse immunoglobulin G (IgG) (Santa Cruz Biotechnology Inc, Santa Cruz, CA, USA). After further washing, the immunoreactive proteins were revealed using the DAB as substrate.

2.5.8 Statistical analysis

Data were compared using independent two sample't' test and chi-square test, as applicable. Ky Plot version 2.0 beta 13 software and Graphpad Prism Software were used for this purpose. Statistical significance was defined as p≤0.05.

3. Result

The clinical characteristics such as age, BMI, endometrial thickness, serum estrogen and progesterone levels of women participating in this study are summarized in Table I.

Parameters	Endometriosis	Control	P value
Age	29.5±0.61	29.32±0.83	P>0.05
BMI	28.18 ± 0.7	26.51 ± 0.6	P>0.05
Endometrial thickness (cm)	9.25 ± 0.25	8.25 ± 0.41	P>0.05
Serum estrogen level (pg/ml)	258.5 ± 13.83	193.6 ± 14.66	P≤0.05
Serum progesterone level (ng/ml)	12.39 ± 1.28	26.43 ± 2	P≤0.05

(Mean ± SEM)

Table 1.

Low levels of immunoreactivity of the endometrial receptivity markers including $\alpha_v\beta_3$ integrin, LIF, L-selectin ligands (MECA-79) and Muc-1 were observed in women with endometriosis in contrast to strong immunoreactivity of controls. In addition, mean expression of these molecular markers detected by flow cytometric analysis shows a significantly lower expression both by the stromal and epithelial cells in women with endometriosis as compared to controls.

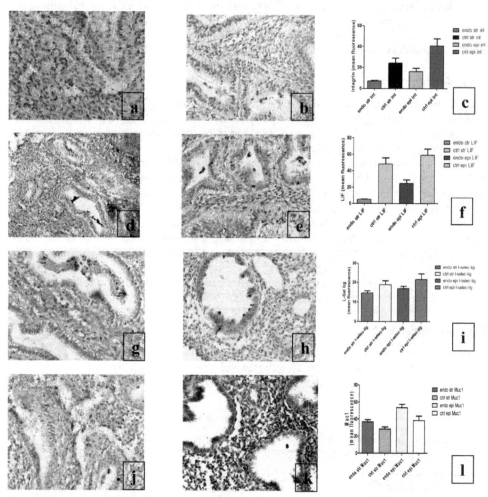

Fig. 1. Immunohistological images of different biochemical markers expression.
a. $\alpha_v\beta_3$ integrins in control **b**. $\alpha_v\beta_3$ integrins in women with endometriosis **c**. Graphical representation of $\alpha_v\beta_3$ integrin expression in the stromal and epithelial cells of endometrial tissues in endometriosis and control **d**. LIF in control **e**. LIF in women with endometriosis **f**. Graphical representation of LIF expression in the stromal and epithelial cells of endometrial tissues in endometriosis and control **g**. L-selectin ligand in control **h**. L-selectin ligand in women with endometriosis **i**. Graphical representation of L-selectin ligand expression in the stromal and epithelial cells of endometrial tissues in endometriosis and control **j**. Muc1 in control **k**. Muc1 in women with endometriosis **l**. Graphical representation of Muc1 expression in the stromal and epithelial cells of endometrial tissues in endometriosis and control.

Further, few poorly developed pinopodes were seen in women with endometriosis as compared to controls, which showed abundant well formed pinopodes (Figure 2, 3 and 4).

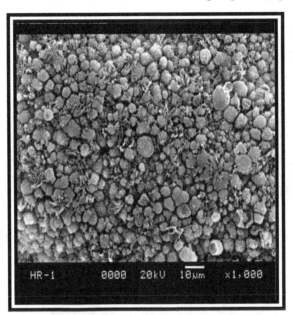

Fig. 2. Well developed pinopodes in control

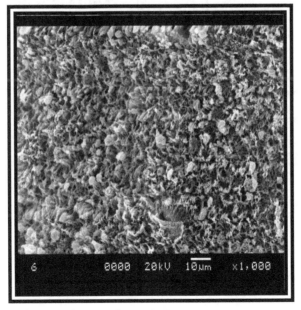

Fig. 3. Poorly developed pinopodes in endometriosis

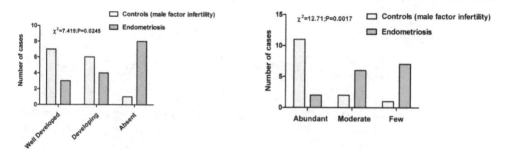

Fig. 4. Graphical representation of pinopode expression in the endometrial tissues in endometriosis and controls.

A significant increase in endometrial MMP-2, -9 and decrease in TIMP-1 and -2 expressions, were observed in women with endometriosis when compared to controls. Further, the endometrial expression of COX-2 was observed to be higher in women with endometriosis when compared with controls.

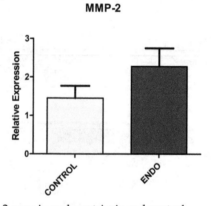

Fig. 5. Expression of MMP-2 gene in endometriosis and control

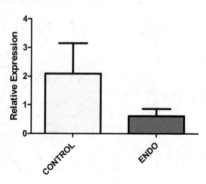

Fig. 6. Expression of TIMP-2 gene in endometriosis and control

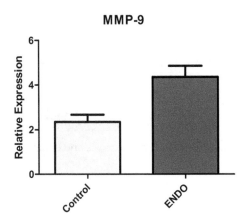

Fig. 7. Expression of MMP-9 gene in endometriosis and control

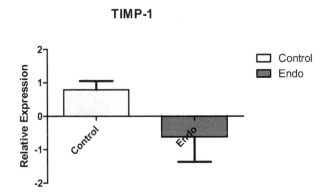

Fig. 8. Expression of TIMP-2 gene in endometriosis and control

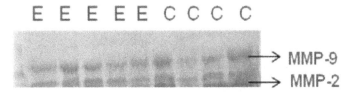

Fig. 9. Expression of MMP-2 and -9 in endometriosis and control

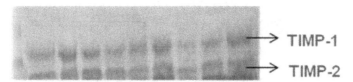

Fig. 10. Expression of TIMP-1 and -2 in endometriosis and control

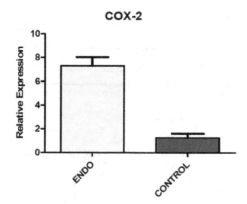

Fig. 11. Expression of COX-2 gene in endometriosis and control

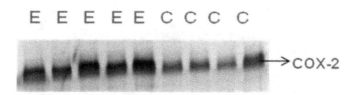

Fig. 12. Expression of COX-2 in endometriosis and control

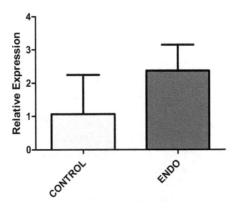

Fig. 13. Expression of VEGFR-1 gene in endometriosis and controls

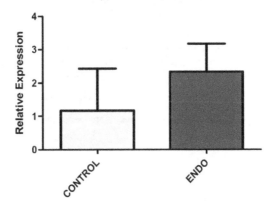

Fig. 14. Expression of VEGFR-2 gene in endometriosis and controls

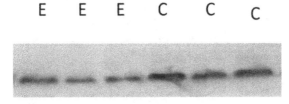

Fig. 15. Expression of endometrial VEGF in endometriotic women and control

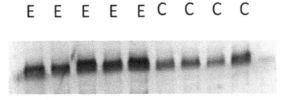

Fig. 16. Expression of endometrial VEGFR in endometriotic women and control

Endometrial expression of VEGF and its receptors VEGFR1 and VEGFR2 were observed to be lower and higher respectively in women with endometriosis when compared with controls.

4. Proposed molecular mechanism for implantation failure in endometriosis and future treatment strategies

In the present study, a hypothesis correlating various factors responsible for implantation failure in endometriosis is proposed (Figure 16). It is well established that endometriosis is an estrogen-dependent disorder. As mentioned earlier, estrogen regulates the expression of MMP-2 and MMP-9 in matrix turnover and VEGF mediated angiogenic activities in various physiological and pathological conditions. Based on our findings, we hypothesize that dysregulation of sex steroids induces over-expression of COX-2 in the endometrium of women with endometriosis. This, in turn, affects endometrial remodelling by up-regulating the expression of MMP-2 and -9, the major molecules responsible for matrix degradation and also increases the expression of VEGF and its receptors, considered to be key angiogenic molecules. This hypothesis is further evidenced by abnormal expression of implantation markers in these women suggesting poor endometrial receptivity and high rate of implantation failure. Molecules which can effectively control excessive endometrial matrix degradation by inhibiting over-expression of various factors responsible for matrix turnover and angiogenesis may be considered as a new therapeutic option for the treatment of endometriosis.

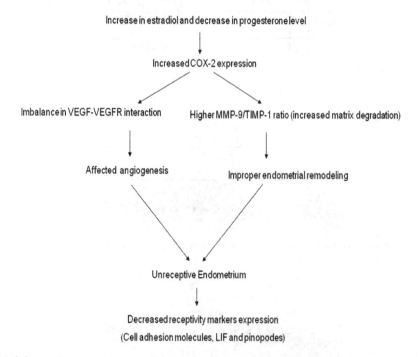

Fig. 16. Schematic representation of the molecular mechanism regulating the process of endometrial receptivity in endometriosis during implantation window

5. References

[1] Au, C.L. & Rogers, P.A. (1993). Immunohistochemical Staining of von Willebrand Factor in Human Endometrium During Normal Menstrual Cycle. *Human Reproduction*, Vol.8, No.1, (January 1993), pp. 17-23, ISSN 1460-2350

[2] Bausero, P.; Cavaille´, F.; Meduri, G.; Freitas, S. & Perrot-Applanat, M. (1998). Paracrine action of vascular endothelial growth factor in the human endometrium: Production and target sites, and hormonal regulation. *Angiogenesis*, Vol.2, No.2, (March 1998), pp. 167–182.

[3] Birkedal-Hansen, H.; Moore, W.G.I.; Bodden, M.K.; Windsor, L.J.; Birkedal-Hansen, B.; DeCarlo, A. *et al.* (1993). Matrix Metalloproteinases: A Review. *Critical Reviews in Oral Biology & Medicine*, Vol.4, No.2, (1993), pp. 197-250.

[4] Charnock-Jones, D.S.; Sharkey, A.M.; Fenwick, P.; & Smith, S.K. (1994). Leukaemia inhibitory factor mRNA concentration peaks in human endometrium at the time of implantation and the blastocyst contains mRNA for the receptor at this time. *Journal of Reproduction and Fertility*, Vol.101, No.2, (July 1994), pp. 421-426.

[5] Charnock-Jones, D.S.; Sharkey, A.M.; Rajput-Williams, J.; Burch, D.; Schofield, J.P.; Fountain, S.A. *et al.* (1993). Identification and localization of alternately spliced mRNAs for vascular endothelial growth factor in human uterus and estrogen regulation in endometrial carcinoma cell lines. *Biology of Reproduction*, Vol.48, No.5, (May 1993), pp. 1120-1128.

[6] Curry, T.E. Jr.; Osteen, K.G. (2003) The matrix metalloproteinase system: changes, regulation, and impact throughout the ovarian and uterine reproductive cycle. Endocrine Reviews, Vol.24, No.4, (Aug 2003), pp. 428-465.

[7] Ferrara, N.; Davis-Smyth, T. (1997) The biology of vascular endothelial growth factor. Endocrine Reviews, Vol.18, No.1, (Feb 1997), pp. 4-25.

[8] Ferrara, N.; Gerber, H.P.; & LeCouter, J. The biology of VEGF and its receptors. Nat Med 2003;9:669-76.

[9] Friedler S, Zimerman A, Schachter M, Raziel A, Strassburger D, Ron El R. The midluteal decline in serum estradiol levels is drastic but not deleterious for implantation after in vitro fertilization and embryo transfer in patients with normal or high responses. Fertility and Sterility 2005;83:54-60.

[10] Giudice L 1996 The endometrial cycle. In Reproductive Endocrinology, Surgery and Technology, pp 272–300. Eds EY Adashi, JA Rock & Z Rosenwaks. Philadelphia: Lippincolt-Raven Publishers.

[11] Perrot-Applanat M 2000 Hormonal regulation of vascular cell function: angiogenesis. In Encyclopedic Reference of Vascular Biology and Pathology pp 157–162. Ed A Bikfalvi. Heidelberg: Springer Verlag.

[12] Genbacev OD, Prakobphol A, Foulk RA, Krtolica AR, Ilic D, Singer MS. Trophoblast L-Selectin-Mediated Adhesion at the Maternal-Fetal Interface. Science 2003;299:405-8.

[13] Gendler SJ, Lancaster CA, Taylor-Papadimitriou J, Duhig T, Peat N, Burchell J. Molecular cloning and expression of human tumor-associated polymorphic epithelial mucin. J Biol Chem 1990;265:15286-93.

[14] Gipson IK, Ho SB, Spurr-Michaud SJ, Tisdale AS, Zhan Q, Torlakovic E. Mucin genes expressed by human female reproductive tract epithelia. Biol Reprod 1997;56:999-1011.

[15] Groothuis PG, Dassen HH, Romano A, Punyadeera C. Estrogen and the endometrium: lessons learned from gene expression profiling in rodents and human. Hum Reprod Update 2007;13:405-17.

[16] Hilkens J, Ligtenberg MJL, Vos HL, Litvinov SV. Cell membrane-associated mucins and their adhesion-modulating property. Trends in Biochemical Sciences 1992;17:359-63.

[17] Hulboy DL, Rudolph LA, Matrisian LM. Matrix metalloproteinases as mediators of reproductive function. Molecular Human Reproduction 1997;3:27-45.

[18] Hung Yu Ng E, Shu Biu Yeung W, Yee Lan Lau E, Wai Ki So W, Chung Ho P. A rapid decline in serum oestradiol concentrations around the mid-luteal phase had no adverse effect on outcome in 763 assisted reproduction cycles. Human Reproduction 2000;15:1903-8.

[19] Itatsu K, Sasaki M, Yamaguchi J, Ohira S, Ishikawa A, Ikeda H et al. Cyclooxygenase-2 Is Involved in the Up-Regulation of Matrix Metalloproteinase-9 in Cholangiocarcinoma Induced by Tumor Necrosis Factor-{alpha}. Am J Pathol 2009;174:829-41.

[20] Kosmas IP, Kolibianakis EM, Devroey P. Association of estradiol levels on the day of hCG administration and pregnancy achievement in IVF: a systematic review. Hum Reprod 2004;19:2446-53.

[21] Kottur A, Rao K, Srinivas M, Gupta N, Shetty N, Narvekar S. The degree of serum estradiol decline in early and midluteal phase had no adverse effect on IVF/ICSI outcome. J Hum Reprod Sci. 2010 Jan-Apr; 3(1): 25–30.

[22] Kyrou D, Popovic-Todorovic B, Fatemi HM, Bourgain C, Haentjens P, Van Landuyt. L .Does the estradiol level on the day of human chorionic gonadotrophin administration have an impact on pregnancy rates in patients treated with rec-FSH/GnRH antagonist? Human Reproduction 2009;24:2902-9.

[23] Lass A, Weiser W, Munafo A, Loumaye E. Leukemia inhibitory factor in human reproduction. Fertil Steril 2001;76:1091-6.

[24] Lessey BA, Castelbaum AJ, Sawin SW, Buck CA, Schinnar R, Bilker W . Aberrant integrin expression in the endometrium of women with endometriosis. J Clin Endocrinol Metab 1994;79:643-9.

[25] Li Y, Pu D, Li Y. The expression of cyclooxygenase-2 in cervical cancers and Hela cells was regulated by estrogen/progestogen. Journal of Huazhong University of Science and Technology -- Medical Sciences -- 2007;27:457-60.

[26] Lockwood CJ, Krikun G, Koo AB, Kadner S, Schatz F. Differential effects of thrombin and hypoxia on endometrial stromal and glandular epithelial cell vascular endothelial growth factor expression. J Clin Endocrinol Metab 2002;87:4280-6.

[27] McIntush EW, Smith MF. Matrix metalloproteinases and tissue inhibitors of metalloproteinases in ovarian function. Rev Reprod 1998;3:23-30.

[28] Nayak NR, Brenner RM. Vascular proliferation and vascular endothelial growth factor expression in the rhesus macaque endometrium. J Clin Endocrinol Metab 2002;87:1845-55.

[29] Okada H, Sanezumi M, Nakajima T, Okada S, Yasuda K, Kanzaki H. Rapid down-regulation of CD63 transcription by progesterone in human endometrial stromal cells. Mol Hum Reprod 1999;5:554-8.

[30] Ota H, Igarashi S, Tanaka T. Morphometric evaluation of stromal vascularization in the endometrium in adenomyosis. Hum Reprod 1998;13:715-9.

[31] Perrot-Applanat M, Ancelin M, Buteau-Lozano H, Meduri G, Bausero P. Ovarian steroids in endometrial angiogenesis. Steroids 2000;65:599-603.

[32] Popovici RM, Irwin JC, Giaccia AJ, Giudice LC. Hypoxia and cAMP Stimulate Vascular Endothelial Growth Factor (VEGF) in Human Endometrial Stromal Cells: Potential Relevance to Menstruation and Endometrial Regeneration. Journal of Clinical Endocrinology & Metabolism 1999;84:2245.

[33] Rogers PA, Au CL, Affandi B. Endometrial microvascular density during the normal menstrual cycle and following exposure to long-term levonorgestrel. Hum Reprod 1993;8:1396-404.

[34] Salata IM, Stojanovic N, Cajdler-Åuba A, Lewandowski KC, LewiÅ„ski A. Gelatinase A (MM-2), gelatinase B (MMP-9) and their inhibitors (TIMP 1, TIMP-2) in serum of women with endometriosis: Significant correlation between MMP-2, MMP9 and their inhibitors without difference in levels of matrix metalloproteinases and tissue inhibitors of metalloproteinases in relation to the severity of endometriosis. Gynecological Endocrinology 2008;24:326-30.

[35] Sharara FI, McClamrock HD. Ratio of oestradiol concentration on the day of human chorionic gonadotrophin administration to mid-luteal oestradiol concentration is predictive of in-vitro fertilization outcome. Human Reproduction 1999;14:2777-82.

[36] Shifren JL, Tseng JF, Zaloudek CJ, Ryan IP, Meng YG, Ferrara N et al. Ovarian steroid regulation of vascular endothelial growth factor in the human endometrium: implications for angiogenesis during the menstrual cycle and in the pathogenesis of endometriosis. J Clin Endocrinol Metab 1996;81:3112-8.

[37] SimÃ³n C, Cano F, Valbuena D, RemohÃ- J, Pellicer A. Implantation: Clinical evidence for a detrimental effect on uterine receptivity of high serum oestradiol concentrations in high and normal responder patients. Human Reproduction 1995;10:2432-7.

[38] Smith SK. Angiogenesis, vascular endothelial growth factor and the endometrium. Hum Reprod Update 1998;4:509-19.

[39] Sugino N, Kashida S, Karube-Harada A, Takiguchi S, Kato H. Expression of vascular endothelial growth factor (VEGF) and its receptors in human endometrium throughout the menstrual cycle and in early pregnancy. Reproduction 2002;123:379-87.

[40] Torry DS, Torry RJ. Angiogenesis and the expression of vascular endothelial growth factor in endometrium and placenta. Am J Reprod Immunol 1997;37:21-9.

[41] Valbuena D, Martin J, de Pablo JL, Remohí J, Pellicer A, Simón C. Increasing levels of estradiol are deleterious to embryonic implantation because they directly affect the embryo. Fertility and Sterility 2001;76:962-8.

[42] Wang Y, Zhao AM, Lin QD. Role of cyclooxygenase-2 signalling pathway dysfunction in unexplained recurrent spontaneous abortion. *Chin Med J (Engl)* 2010;123:1543-1547.1

[43] Wesseling J, van der Valk SW, Hilkens J. A mechanism for inhibition of E-cadherin-mediated cell-cell adhesion by the membrane-associated mucin episialin/MUC1. Mol Biol Cell 1996;7:565-77.

[44] Xiong B, Sun TJ, Hu WD, Cheng FL, Mao M, Zhou YF. Expression of cyclooxygenase-2 in colorectal cancer and its clinical significance. World J Gastroenterol 2005;11:1105-8.

5

Analysis of Differential Genes of Uyghur Women with Endometriosis in Xinjiang

Aixingzi Aili, Ding Yan, Hu Wenjing, Yang Xinhua and Hanikezi Tuerxun
Xinjiang Medical University,
China

1. Introduction

Endometriosis (EM) is a common and important health problem, it is estimated to be present in 10%-15% of women in the reproductive age group and 25%-35% of infertile women. In the First Affiliated Hospital of Xinjiang Medical University in China, 447 cases primaily diagnosed with surgically confirmed endometriosis between January 2000 to September 2005, among them 349 cases of endometriosis were Han Chinese (78.1%) and 69 cases Uyghur women with endometriosis (15.3%).

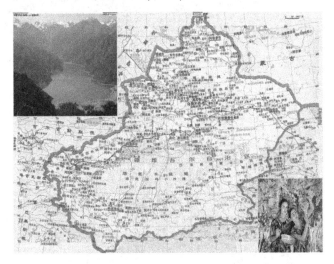

Fig. 1.

Xinjiang is the biggest province of China inhabited by ethnic minorities in which Uyghur people are accounted for more than 40% of the total population. In recent years, the number of the Uyghur women with endometriosis have been increased in Xinjiang, however still clearly less than Han chinese with endometriosis. The data from pathology deparment of the First Affiliated Hospital of Xinjiang Medical University between 1992 and 1996 showed that there were only three Uyghur women with endometriosis (5.76%) among 52 cases. Between 2000 and 2001, only 4 Uyghur women with endometriosis (3.1%) among 128 patients. Between 2003 and 2010, there were 73 Uyghur women (13.45%) with endometriosis in 565 cases. In Kashi, the Uyghur is occupied more than 80% of population. In the last 8 years, there were only 16 Uyghur women with endometriosis among 600 cases of endometriosis in People's Hospital of Kashi. It was demonstrated that the number of Uyghur women with endometriosis dramaticaly lower than Han chinese.

We performed AtlasTMcDNA Expression Arrays (Clontech # 7854-1) cDNA microarray (containing 22,000. DNA)to compare the differential expression genes between ectopic endometrium of Uyghur and Han chinese women with endometriosis. Our study aimed to explore the molecular pathogenesis of endometriosis ethnic differences, so as to determine the cause of endometriosis of Uyghur women in Xinjiang.

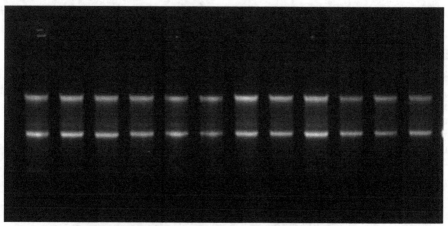

Fig. 2. Total RNA results.

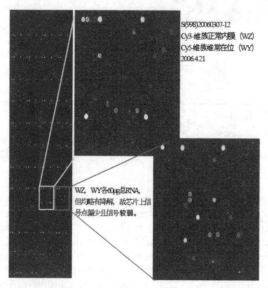

Fig. 3. Uyghur with and without endometriosis ectopic endometriosis hybrid.

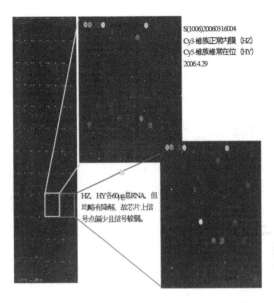

Fig. 4. Han with and without endometriosis ectopic endometriosis hybrid.

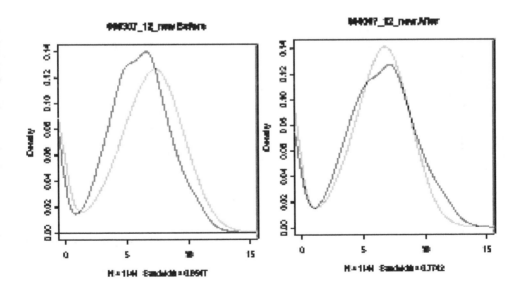

Fig. 5. Uyghur with and without endometriosis ectopic endometriosis hybrid before and after correction signal strength distribution.

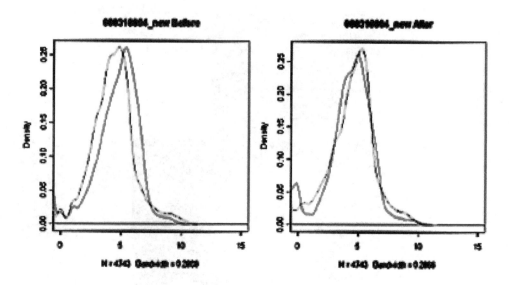

Fig. 6. Han with and without endometriosis ectopic endometriosis hybrid before and after correction signal strength distribution.

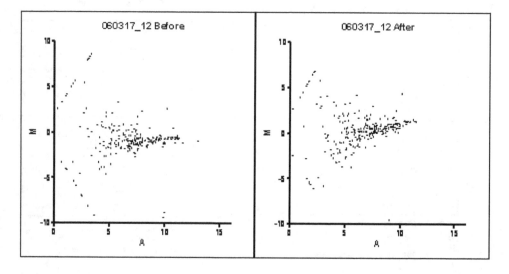

Fig. 7. Uyghur with and without endometriosis ectopic endometriosis hybrid before and after correction signal scatter.

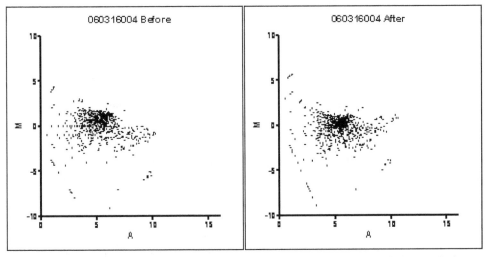

Fig. 8. Han with and without endometriosis ectopic endometriosis hybrid before and after correction signal scatter.

ID	Name	Cy5/Cy	Description
4340	FOS	3.649786	V-fos FBJ murine osteosarcoma viral oncogene homolog
7224	DCN	2.250099	Decorin
10599	VIM	1.629836	Vimentin
1900	GNG5	1.211619	Guanine nucleotide binding protein (G protein), gamma 5
1527	XCL1	1.169442	Small inducible cytokine subfamily C, mendometriosisber 1 (lymphotactin)
13167	IGFBP7	1.114798	Insulin-like growth factor binding protein 7
1651	RPS23	1.093641	Ribosomal protein S23
22665	TIMP3	-1.15294	Tissue inhibitor of metalloproteinase 3
13265	COL3A1	-1.55893	Collagen, type III, alpha 1 (Ehlers-Danlos syndrome type IV, autosomal dominant)
21389	RPL29	-1.63396	Ribosomal protein L29
8626	GAPD	-2.01536	Glyceraldehyde-3-phosphate dehydrogenase
22689	GAPD	-2.30404	Glyceraldehyde-3-phosphate dehydrogenase
22785	GAPD	-2.71698	Glyceraldehyde-3-phosphate dehydrogenase

Table 1. Uyghur with and without endometriosis ectopic endometriosis differential genes.

ID	Name	Rate of Cy5/Cy3	Description
18428	FTL	4.340706	ESTs, Weakly similar to FRHUL ferritin light chain [H.sapiens]
8586	APOE	3.768085	Apolipoprotein E
7998	CD74	3.623251	CD74 antigen (invariant polypeptide of major histocompatibility complex, class II antigen-associated
21034	CTSD	2.992721	Cathepsin D (lysosomal aspartyl protease)
20900	IGL@	2.941947	H.sapiens mRNA for IgG lambda light chain V-J-C region (clone Tgl9)
18699	BIN3	3.235432	Bridging integrator 3
10633	CTSB	2.736133	Cathepsin B
16743	IGKV1-9	2.482954	Immunoglobulin kappa variable 1-9
10901	IGHG3	2.24961	Immunoglobulin heavy constant gamma 3 (G3m marker)
17716	ZFHXI B	2.221742	Zinc finger homeobox 1 b
15732	ACTA2	1.939791	Actin, alpha 2, smooth muscle, aorta
6876	HLA-G	1.795164	HLA-G histocompatibility antigen, class I, G
9464	HLA-A	1.617767	Major histocompatibility complex, class I, A
12611	ITM2C	1.60875	Integral mendometriosisbrane protein 3
9202	DLGAP4	1.56221	KIAA0964 protein
6875	WNT7A	1.55996	Wingless-type MMTV integration site family, mendometriosisber 7A
6494	FTH1	1.55145	Ferritin, heavy polypeptide 1
6952	TMSB10	1.539032	Thymosin, beta 10
22794	ACTB	1.51553	Actin, beta
22769	ACTB	1.495315	Actin, beta
10474	FLJ14950	1.489821	Hypothetical protein FLJ14950
13167	IGFBP7	1.486395	Insulin-like growth factor binding protein 7
18071	HUMMHC W1A	1.460991	Cw1 antigen
22698	ACTB	1.45868	Actin, beta
12651	SPARC	1.441213	Secreted protein, acidic, cysteine-rich (osteonectin)
22696	RPL5	1.421712	Ribosomal protein L5
13180	LOC51237	1.416254	Hypothetical protein
14701	HSU79274	1.391079	Protein predicted by clone 23733
22793	ACTB	1.374773	Actin, beta
5712	GPX3	1.370492	Glutathione peroxidase 3(plasma)
22985	ACTB	1.342603	Actin, beta
22674	ACTB	1.333726	Actin, beta
22697	ACTB	1.33342	Actin, beta
21176	KPT13	1.327325	Keratin 13
22889	ACTB	1.325337	Actin, beta
22700	CYC1	1.325323	Cytochrome c-1
23193	LOC389643	1.323453	LOC389643

Table 2. Han with and without endometriosis ectopic endometriosis differential genes.

ID	Name	Rate of Cy5/Cy3	Description
9988	ACTB	1.293784	Actin, beta
20299	IL1 RN	1.283803	Interleukin 1 receptor antagonist
16687	TP73	1.277275	Tumor protein p73
22986	ACTB	1.267406	Actin, beta
22770	ACTB	1.258614	Actin, beta
10599	VIM	1.251847	Vimentin
22865	ACTB	1.233357	Actin, beta
22345	LOC440552	1.232367	similar to OK/SW-CL.16
8173	MARK2	1.227909	ELKL motif kinase
22962	ACTB	1.219306	Actin, beta
21216	SLPI	1.215856	Secretory leukocyte protease inhibitor
22690	ANKT	1.213863	Nucleolar protein
23200	LOC389622	1.212664	LOC389622
22961	ACTB	1.212137	Actin, beta
22673	ACTB	1.210056	Actin, beta
22890	ACTB	1.208872	Actin, beta
19718	SULT1C2	1.207869	Sulfotransferase family, cytosolic, 1C, mendometriosisber 2
12903	HSPA5BP1	1.179906	Hypothetical protein FLJ20539
22785	PDGFRA	1.159421	Platelet-derives growth factor receptor
1900	GNG5	1.125384	Guanine nucleotide binding protein (G protein), gamma 5
20231	SERF2	1.112907	Small EDRK-rich factor 2
15491	ZNF14	1.104864	Zinc finger protein 14 (KOX 6)
9735	KIAA0635	1.100348	Hypothetical protein FLJ13621
16540	CDW92	1.092801	CDw92 antigen
22762	COPEB	1.08944	Core promoterelendometriosisent binding protein
22866	ACTB	1.083347	Actin, beta
8626	GPX3	1.078504	Glutathione peroxidase 3(plasma)
1401	ELAVL3	1.077059	ELAV (endometriosisbryonic lethal, abnormal vision, Drosophila)-like 3 (Hu antigen C)
19581	GNG5	1.057676	Guanine nucleotide binding protein (G protein), gamma 5
7186	ID3	1.057184	Inhibitor of DNA binding 3, dominant negative helix-loop-helix protein
17362	FKBP14	1.036957	Hypothetical protein FLJ20731
9824	MTBP	1.030879	Mdm2, transformed 3T3 cell double minute 2, p53 binding protein (mouse) binding protein, 104kD
8364	ARHGDIA	1.029915	Rho GDP dissociation inhibitor (GDI) alpha
21961	RPS23	1.025033	Ribosomal protein S23
1580	NELF	1.017617	DKFZP586J1624 protein
22665	GAPD	-1.003765	Glyceraldehyde-3-phosphate dehydrogenase
22761	GAPD	-1.001544	Glyceraldehyde-3-phosphate dehydrogenase
17133	GAPD	-4.29046	Glyceraldehyde-3-phosphate dehydrogenase

Table 2. Han with and without endometriosis ectopic endometriosis differential genes. (Continuation)

ID	Name	Rate of Cy5/Cy3	Description
7979	PAEP	-5.57639	Progestagen-associated endometrial protein (placental protein 14, pregnancy-associated endometrial a
1813	TIMP3	-2.748361	Tissue inhibitor of metalloproteinase 3 (erythroid potentiating activity, collagenase inhibitor)

Table 2. Han with and without endometriosis ectopic endometriosis differential genes. (Continuation)

2. The incidence of endometriosis of Uyghur ethnic group in Xinjiang

The incidence of endometriosis has no precise information. Researchs have found that Asian women with endometriosis have a higher prevalence, and its disease risk :OR:8.6(95%CI ll.4—20.7). There was an exploratory study suggested that there might be an associated risk of endometriosis for those women who have worked as a flight attendant, service station attendant, or health worker, particularly a nurse. But they have not been reported the correlation between nationality, religion and other factors with endometriosis.

Clinical and epidemiological survey found that endometriosis has a genetic predisposition and significant family aggregation, and it loss of heterozygosity of 40% -70%. Dingyan(researcher in Xinjiang) found that no evidence was found to suggest an association between GSTM1-null genotype and endometriosis in the Hans chinese and Uyghurs. An association was found between GSTT1 -null genotype and endometriosis in the Hans chinese, but not in the Uyghurs. The two ethnic groups have different genetic predisposing factors to the development of endometriosis. There were significant difference in the frequencies of these two points among the Han chinese, European and Uyghur in Xinjiang. In Uyghur the distribution of CYP 1 A 1 /MspI genotypes were different from Han chinese and European.

3. The spectrum of microarray applications on endometriosis

A large number of microarray gene-specific cDNA are fixed on a glass or silica using the hybridization principles to detect the mRNA of the different sources. This study shows the different organization, different cells and tissues in different developmental stages that have differentially expressed genes. Development of molecular mechanisms provide theoretical basis for gene diagnosis and treatment of cutting-edge biotechnology. The theory proposed by Sampson in 1927 suggests that endometrial tissue is released into the peritoneal cavity via retrograde menstruation. The shed tissue then implants and grows ectopically. This theory is supported by the fact that up to 76% -90% of women experience retrograde menstruation ; and yet, endometriosis only affects 10% -15% of women. Reference to foreign literature, different individuals sample of patient with endometriosis geometric mixed, different individuals sample of patient without endometriosis geometric mixed, to eliminate non-specific genetic differences between individuals, and search for specific associated genes with endometriosis. By the gene microarray expression profiling 22,000 points compare ectopic endometrium and normal ectopic endometrial of the Uyghur and Han chinese with endometriosis, 11 differential genes expressed in ectopic endometrium were screened out between Uyhgur women with or without endometriosis respectively, FOS, DCN, VIN, GNGS, XCL 1, IGFBP7, PRS23, TIMP3, COL3A1, PRL29, GAPD; GAPD expression in the three loci, including FOS, DCN, VIN, GNGS, XCL1, IGFBP7, PRS23 were up-regulated, and TIMP3, COL3A1, PRL29, GAPD were down-regulated. The Han chinese group were significantly different genes, 58 of which TIMP3, PAEP, GADP were down-regulated, but GADP expressed in three loci shows different range. And from a different CD74, ACTA2, GPX3 and other 55 genes were upregulated, ACTB appear in 17 loci, GNGS appear in two loci. The same genes difference between the two groups is VIM, GNGS, PRS23, GAPD, TIMP3, including GAPD, TIMP3 are down-regulated. We get different genes according to their main function and are divided into the following categories: immune-related genes,proto-oncogenes and tumor suppressor genes,cell receptor,ion channels and transport protein; cytoskeleton and sports-related protein, apoptosis-related protein; DNA synthesis and repair, recombinant protein, DNA binding, transcription and transcription factors,cell signaling and transmission white and some unknown functional genes.

4. The possible role of clinically relevant different gene in endometriosis pathogenesis

The difference in the screened genes, tissue inhibitor of metalloproteinase 3 (TIMP-3) both in the Han chinese and Uyghur with endometriosis were down-regulated. The study of Zhou Honghui found that TIMP-3 down-regulation is remarkable in the secretory phase than proliferative phase. TIMP is a metalloproteinase (MMPs) inhibitors by the endometrial cells of MMPs which plays an important role in the invasion of the peritoneum and other connective tissue. Increased endometrial MMPs and TIMP down-regulation with the development of endometriosis is closely related. Because of TIMP up-regulation and MMPs down-reglation, ectopic endometrial of endometriosis is more invasive than normal force, and develop to the peritoneal endometriotic lesions.Angiogenesis is considered as a major process in the pathogenesis of endometriosis. Many factors are involved in this complex mechanism, and the vascular endothelial growth factor (VEGF) is an important mediator of angiogenesis; it is a potent endothelial cell mitogen, morphogen, and vascular permeability-inducing agent. VEGF binds to either of two tyrosine kinase receptors, the fm5-like tyrosine kinase (flt) and the kinase domain receptor (KDR or Flk-1). Peritoneal endometriotic lesions with high proliferative activity are also accompanied by high angiogenic activity, as reflected by higher expression of VEGF-A in stroma and glandular epithelium and VEGFR-2 in blood vessels. In our recent study, we showed that the vascular density and the expression of VEGF and its receptor VEGFR-2 (Flk-1) are significantly higher in deeply infiltrating endometriosis affecting the ovary, bladder and mainly the rectosigmoid, compared with the ectopic endometrium.

Controlled clinical analyses of angiogenesis in human endometriotic lesions are limited, because it is not possible to monitor the lesions without repeated laparoscopies. Thus, research into the fundamental mechanisms by which menstrual endometrium adheres, invades and establishes a functional vasculature to persist in an ectopic site, as well as the development of new therapeutical approaches, is best performed in experimental animal models. In contrast to humans and non-human primates, estrous animals do not shed their endometrial tissue and therefore do not develop endometriosis spontaneously. However, endometriosis can be induced by transplanting endometrial tissue to ectopic sites, and the establishment of an experimental model of endometriosis may be a good way to study the endometriosis angiogenesis process, and allow evaluation of the balance of the many factors involved.

This study by glyceraldehyde 3-phosphate dehydrogenase (GAPD) gene in Han chinese and Uyghurs with endometriosis group are down-regulated, GAPD genes are housekeeping gene family, Gene bank No. NM-002046, is a basic enzyme in the human body.It is a key enzyme of a series of biochemical reactions of the glycolysis, which generate ATP for the source of human cells energy, a variety of cells are present in the body, involved in glucose metabolism in glycolysis, in 12p13.

In Han and Uyghur groups the same set of common up-regulated genes are GNGS, VIM and PRS23. Abundance or localization changes in endometrial tissue were validated by immunohistochemistry and Western blotting. In addition, multiple charge and size isoforms were observed for VIM in endometriosis patients that was below the level of detection in healthy women.

Our experiment confirmed endometriosis may be related to multiple factors similar as diabetes, asthma, cancer-related disease, genetics and aberrant regulation in the endometrium and endometriotic. Lower different genes expression on Uyghur women with endometriosis compared to Han Chinese women with endometriosis may be the essential factor for relatively lower incidence of endometriosis on Uyghur women. Most genes we found on the endometrium of both Uyghur and Han Chinese women with endometriosis were the cytoskeleton, adhesion, invaded and immune related gene,patially explained the mechanism of malignant biological behaviors.

5. References

[1] O Down MJ, Philipp EE. The history of obstetrics and gynecology. New York: The Parthenon Publishing group, 2000,523.

[2] Jinghe Lang. The new progress on endometriosis research, Chinese journal of obstetrics and gynecology. 2005, 40:3-4.

[3] Stephen K, Simon B, Daniel EW. Genetics and infertility II affected sib-pair analysis in endometriosis. Hum Reprod Update, 2001,7(4): 411-418

[4] Eskenazi B, Warner ML. Epidemiology of endometriosis. Obstet Gynecol Clin North Am, 1997,24(2):235-258.

[5] Zondervan KT. The genetic basis of endometriosis. Curr Opin Obstet Gynecol, 2001,13(3):309-314.

[6] Qiaozhi Lin, Baozheng Wu .Endometriosis. Qiaozhi Lin's gynecology oncology. Beijin, People's Publishing House, the third edition, 2000,697-713.

[7] Eskenazi B, Warner ML. Epidemiology of endometriosis. Obstet Gynecol Clin North Am, 1997,24(2):235-258.

[8] Yan Ding, Zhifang Chen, Jianyong ChenThe Study on the differential genes expression on women with endometriosis in Xinjiang. Chinese journal of obstetrics and gynecology., 2004,39(2):101-104.

[9] Hawkins T, Venkatesh B, Rokhsar D, et al. Whole-genome shotgun assembly and analysis of the genome of Fugu rubripes. Science, 2002, 297:1301-1310.

[10] Jinghe Lang. The basic and clinical research of endometriosis. Beijin; Beijing union medical university press , 2003:35-50.

[11] Yali Li, Huilan Zhang. Endometriosis [J]. Chin J Pract Gynecol Obstet, 2002,18:131-172.

[12] Jane M, Borthwick D, Stephen C, et al. Determination of the trans- cript profile of human endometrium[J]. Molecular Human Reproduc- tion, 2003,9:19-33.

[13] Honghui Zhou, Yali Li, Jie Li, Screening differential genes expression associated with endometriosis with expression gene chip. Progress in Obstetrics and Gynecology, 2004, 13(6):406-409.

[14] Majid MA, Smith VA, Rasty DL, et al. Adenovirus mediated gene dilivery of tissue inhibitor of metalloproteinases-3 induces death in retinal pigment epithilial cells[J]. Br J Ophthalmol, 2002,86:97-101.

[15] Gao Y, Zhou S, Jiang W, et al. Effects of ganopoly on the immune functions in advanced-stage cancer patients. Immunol Invest, 2003,32 (3):201-215.

[16] Hsu MJ, Lee SS, Lee ST, et al. Signaling mechanisms of enhanced neutrophil phagocytosis and chemotaxis by the polysaccharide purified from Ganoderma lucidum. Br J Pharmacol, 2003,139(2):289- 298.

[17] Liu B, Aronson N, N Jr. Structure of human G protein gene GNG5[J]. Biochem Biophys Res Commun, 1998,251:88.

[18] Gough NR, Adler ENDOMETRIOSIS, Ray LB. Focus issue:targeting signaling pathways for drug discovery[J]. Sci STKE, 2004,(225):EG5.

[19] Perrenu J, Lilienlxaum A, Vasseur M, et al. Nucleotide Sequence of the vimentin gene [J]. 1988,62(1):7.

[20] Ferram S, Cartnizzare A, Battin R, et al. Human vimentin is readed on the short arm of chromosome 10[J]. Am J Hum Gene, 1987,4(14): 616.

[21] Nikcolic B, Nully E B, Mir H et al. Basic acid residue cluster within nuclear targeting sequence is assential for cytoplasma plectin- bimentin network junctions[J]J Cell Biol, 1996,134(6):1455.

[22] Hermann H, Aebi H. Intermediate filaments and their associates: multi-talented structural elements specifying cytoarchitecture and cytodynamics[J]. Curr Opin Cell Biol, 2000,12:79-90.

[23] Quax W, Meera khan P, Quax-jeuken Y. The structure of the vimentin gen[J]. Cell, 1983,35(1)215.

[24] Mingtong Xu,Lin Lv, Zhinu Zhong, People leptin gene cloning and sequence determined [J]. Sen University of Medical Sciences. 2000,21(2):104.

[25] Zoppi N, Oardella R, De Paepe A, et al. Human fibroblasts with mutations in COL5A1 and COL3A1 genes do not organize collagens and fibronectin in the extracellular matrix, down—regulate alpha2beta1 integrin, and recruit alphavbeta3 instead of alphasbeta1 integrin[J]. J Biol Chem, 2004,279(18):18157-18168.

[26] Thomas EJ, Campbell G. Molecular genetic defects in endometriosis. Gynecol Obstet Invest, 2000,50(supl 1)44-50.

[27] Sendometriosisino C, Sendometriosisino A, Pietra G, et al. Role of major histocompatibility complex class I expression and natural killer-like T cells in the genetic control of endometriosis. Fertil Steril, 1995,64:909-916.

[28] Xin Wang, Chunyu Liu, Endometriosis [J]. People leptin gene cloning and sequence determined , 2002,37(6):346- 348.

6

Endometriosis and Infertility: The Role of Oxidative Stress

Ionara Barcelos[1] and Paula Navarro[2]
[1]University of West Parana,
Da Vinci - Reproductive Medicine,
[2]University of Sao Paulo,
University of Sao Paulo - Ribeirao Preto,
Brazil

1. Introduction

Several reports have supported the concept of reduced fecundity in women with endometriosis (Garrido et al., 2002; 2000). Contradictory data have been reported for in vitro fertilization (IVF) outcomes in patients with endometriosis (Garrido et al., 2002; Garcia-Velasco & Arici, 1999; Kumbak et al., 2008; Fernando et al., 2008). Some studies suggest lower fertilization, implantation, and pregnancy rates in women with endometriosis (Barnhardt et al., 2002; Al-Fadhli et al., 2006), possibly owing to impaired oocyte quality with consequent poor embryo quality, or to endometrial defects or defective interactions between the endometrium and the embryo (Kumbak et al., 2008, Brizek et al., 1995; Pellicer et al., 1995).

Oocyte quality depends on proper cytoplasmic and nuclear maturation (Kim et al., 1998), with the latter requiring the presence of normal cell spindles that guide chromosome segregation during meiosis (Wang & Keefe, 2002; Mandelbaum et al., 2004; De Santis et al., 2005; Volarcik et al., 1998; Van Blerkom & Davis, 2001). The cell spindle of the oocyte is extremely sensitive to several factors, including oxidative stress (Liu et al., 2003; Navarro et al., 2004; 2006), which might be involved in the etiopathogenesis of infertility related to endometriosis (Campos Petean et al, 2008; Mansour et al, 2009; Jozwik et al., 1999; Carbone et al., 2003).

The oxidative balance of the reproductive female tract depends on some types of free radicals and on different antioxidant mechanisms that neutralize them. There are two major groups of free radicals: reactive oxygen species and reactive nitrogen species.

2. Reactive Oxygen Species (ROS)

The ROS have physiological and pathological functions in the female reproductive tract. Fertility problems related to ROS have etiopathogenic factors in common (Agarwal et al., 2005). These reactive species are generated through enzymatic and non-enzymatic organic reactions. Biological reactions, through electron transference or through oxigenase, that use oxygen (O_2) as substrate, generate large amounts of ROS. As the mithocondrial respiratory chain is the major O_2 cell intake system, the majority of ROS are produced by this system under physiological conditions (Fujii et al., 2005). The **superoxide radical (O_2^-)** is formed when electrons leak from the electron transport chain ($O_2 + e^- \rightarrow O_2^-$) (Agarwal et al., 2005). The dismutation of superoxide results in the formation of **hydrogen peroxide (H_2O_2)** (2 O_2^- + 2 $H^+ \rightarrow H_2O_2 + O_2$) (Agarwal et al., 2005). The same can also be generated by reduction of O_2^- ($O_2^- + e^- + 2 H^+ \rightarrow H_2O_2$) (Babior, 1997). The **hidroxyl (OH·) ion** is formed by the acquisition of 1 electron by H_2O_2 ($H_2O_2 + e^- + H^+ \rightarrow OH + H_2O$) (Babior, 1997). The hydroxyl ion is highly reactive and can modify purines and pyrimidines and cause strand breaks resulting in DNA damage (Agarwal et al., 2005).

3. Antioxidants

Under normal conditions, all organisms have enzymatic and non-enzymatic mechanisms capable of neutralizing pro-oxidants species and/or repair damages caused by reactive species, converting them to H_2O, to prevent overproduction. Many antioxidants of low molecular weight such as vitamins and polyphenols are usually found in nutrients, although enzymatic neutralization of reactive species is the most effective mechanism (Agarwal et al., 2005; Fujii et al., 2005).

4. Non-enzymatic antioxidants

Also known as synthetic antioxidants or dietary supplements, this group influences in an exogenous way the antioxidant defense system of the organism. The most common are: vitamins C and E, selenium, zinc, taurine, hypotaurine, glutathione, β-carotene, and carotene.

Vitamin E may block the initiation of lipid peroxidation as well as its propagation phase (Bornoden, 1994).

Glutathione is the major non-protein sulfhydryl component of mammalian cells and has an important role in cellular protection from oxidative stress (Meister, 1983). Glutathione synthesis increases throughout oocyte development and maturation until the periovulatory follicle stage (Perreault et al., 1988). After fertilization, glutathione participates in the sperm decondensation process, while the oocyte activation process occurs, and the sperm head turns into the male pronucleus (Calvin et al., 1986; Perreault et al., 1984, 1988; Yoshida, 1992, 1993). A study performed with bovine oocytes has shown the important role of COCs during the in vitro maturation process. Through gap junctions, cumulus oophorus cells (COCs) might mediate glutathione synthesis by the oocytes, a crucial enzyme for the cytoplasmic and nuclear maturation process. This intimate relation between COCs and oocytes apparently occurs due to the presence of gap junctions (De Matos et al., 1997).

5. Enzymatic antioxidants

The enzymatic defenses responsible for ROS neutralization are mainly represented by superoxide dismutase (SOD), catalase, glutathione peroxidase (GPx), depending or not on selenium and glutathione reductase (GR) (Fujii et al., 2005):

- **Superoxide dismutase (SOD):**

The superoxide anion is produced by a one-electron reduction of an oxygen molecule and initiates a radical chain reaction. It is believed that SOD, which dismutates the superoxide anion to hydrogen peroxide ($2 O_2^- + 2 H^+ \rightarrow H_2O_2 + O_2$), plays a central role in antioxidant reactions. Three isozymes are produced by mammals (Fujii et al., 2005):

- SOD1 encodes Cu,Zn-SOD, which is largely cytosolic;
- SOD2 encodes Mn-SOD, a mitochondrial isoform;
- SOD3, which encodes the extracellular form (EC-SOD), structurally similar to CuZn-SOD.

One of the striking phenotypes of SOD1-deficient mice is female infertility, suggesting a potential role of this enzyme in female fertility. SOD2 is inducible under various oxidative stress and inflammatory conditions. EC-SOD is present at high levels in the epididymis, seminiferous tubules of the testis, as well as the lungs (Fujii et al., 2005).

The presence of SOD was evidenced in human follicular fluid (FF) and the identification of high concentrations of SOD in FF was associated with oocytes that were not fertilized (Sabatini et al., 1999). Data of a recently published study showed that SOD activity decreased with age in women, but increased in women with endometriosis and ovulatory dysfunction (Matos et al., 2009). When the cause of infertility was male factor, the success of ART was associated with increased SOD activity. Variations in SOD activity emphasize the importance of oxidative stress in the oocyte maturation process, and are suggested to be a potential biomarker of ART success (Matos et al., 2009).

A recent study has established a threshold level in FF which ROS may be considered toxic for viable embryo formation and pregnancy outcome. ROS, lipid peroxidation and total antioxidant capacity were estimated. The upper cut-off ROS level beyond which viable embryo formation is not favorable was found to be approximately 107 cps/400 microl FF. This level, determined in women with tubal factor infertility, was further validated in women with endometriosis and PCOS and correlated with fertilization and pregnancy rate and embryo quality (Jana et al., 2010).

- **Peroxidases:**

Catalase exclusively detoxifies hydrogen peroxide and has no requirement for an electron donor **($2 H_2O_2 \rightarrow 2 H_2O + O_2$)**. It plays a role in organs such as the liver, but its specific function in the genital tract is largely unknown (Fujii et al., 2005).

Glutathione is a tripeptidyl molecule and is present in either the reduced (GSH) or the oxidized state (GSSG). It plays pleiotropic roles, which include the maintenance of cells in a reduced state and the formation of conjugates with some harmful endogenous and xenobiotic compounds. In addition, GSH serves as an electron donor for GPx that reduces peroxide **($2GSH + H_2O_2 \rightarrow GSSG + 2 H_2O$)**. At least four selenium-containing GPx isozymes are produced in mammals (Fujii et al., 2005):

The cytosolic form, GPX1, is widely distributed in tissues and has been the most extensively investigated form. However, GPX1-knockout mice show no abnormality in phenotype including reproductive capability (Ho et al., 1997);

- GPX2 encodes a gastrointestinal form, and no specific function for it is known in reproduction
- GPX3 is present in plasma and in epididymal fluid
- GPX4 encodes an isoform that specifically detoxifies phospholipid hydroperoxide and is thus referred to as PhGPx, and is expressed at high levels in the testis. A defect in GPX4 has been suspected to be a cause of male infertility triggered by selenium deficiency, although direct evidence for its requirement is missing (Hansen & Deguchi, 1996).

In a reaction promoted by peroxidase, GSH is oxidized to GSSG. Regeneration of GSH is, therefore, crucial for the ability of cells to fight exposure to oxidant metabolites. GSH levels are maintained by de novo synthesis that is catalyzed by two enzymes, γ- glutamylcysteine synthetase (γ-GCS) and glutathione synthetase (GS). The reduction of GSSG is catalyzed by **glutathione reductase** (GR) using NADPH as an electron donor **(2 GSSG + NADPH + H$^+$ → 2GSH + NADP$^+$)**. GR is also inhibited by compounds produced in response to nitrosative stress, such as nitrosoglutathione. In the female reproductive system, GSH is assumed to play a role by reducing oxidative stress either by direct interaction with ROS, by the **glutathione redox system**, or by donating an electron to GPx (Fujii et al., 2005).

High levels of SeGPx were found in follicles that held oocytes with the potential to be fertilized and lower levels were related to fertilization failure (Paszkowski et al., 1995).

6. Endometriosis and oxidative stress

Some authors have suggested that endometriosis might be associated with oxidative stress (Agarwal et al., 2003; Szczepanska et al., 2003; Gupta et al., 2006). In pelvic endometriosis there might be an activation of macrophages in the peritoneal environment leading to increased production of reactive oxygen and nitrogen species, cytokines, prostaglandins, growth factors and, therefore, oxidative stress generating lipid peroxidation and its degradation products and other products formed by its interactions with low density lipoproteins and other proteins. Peroxidized lipids, when decomposed, generate products such as malondialdehyde (MDA) and could be recognized as foreign bodies, leading to an antigenic response with consequent production of antibodies (Halliwell, 1994; Murphy et al., 1998). This process would induce oxidative damage to red blood cells and to endometrial and peritoneal cells which would stimulate recruitment and activation of a larger number of mononuclear phagocytes, maintaining oxidative damage to the pelvic environment (Van Langendonckt et al., 2002). Oxidative stress compromises mesothelial cells and might induce adhesion sites for endometrial cells, contributing to development and progression of the endometriosis focus (Alpay et al., 2006).

In a recent study by our group, blood samples were collected during the early follicular phase of the menstrual cycle for the analysis of serum MDA, GSH and total hydroxyperoxide levels by spectrophotometry and of vitamin E by high performance liquid chromatography. A positive association between infertility related to endometriosis, advanced disease stage and increased serum hydroxyperoxide levels was demonstrated, suggesting an increased production of reactive species in women with endometriosis. These data, taken together with the reduction of serum vitamin E and GSH levels, suggest the occurrence of systemic oxidative stress in women with infertility associated with endometriosis (Andrade et al., 2010).

The activation of polymorphonuclear leucocytes and macrophages observed in endometriosis patients might be induced by several factors, including damaged red blood cells, apoptotic endometrial cells, cellular debris and some other inflammatory cells. In endometriosis these actions of peritoneal macrophages appear to be stimulated *in vitro* by the immune response or by agents such as α and γ-interferon, increasing inducible nitric oxide synthase (NOS) expression, producing more nitric oxide and nitrite and nitrate compounds (Agarwal et al., 2005). However, we obtained no conclusive data concerning nitric oxide, peroxidized lipids and ROS levels in the peritoneal fluid of patients with and without endometriosis (Agarwal et al., 2003; Amaral et al., 2005).

In women with endometriosis and adenomyosis, we also observe a greater expression of Mn-SOD and CuZn-SOD in the endometrium throughout the menstrual cycle, as well as aberrant expression of GPx and xanthine peroxidase (XO), in topic and ectopic endometrium. SOD activity seems to be significantly higher in the ectopic endometrium of endometriomas than in the topic endometrium (Alpay et al., 2006). However, this increase in the expression of antioxidant enzymes in the topic and ectopic endometrium of endometriosis patients could be a primary event or secondary to an increase of ROS, which needs to be evaluated. If, on the one hand, we have no conclusive data concerning the pattern of expression of the most important oxidant and antioxidant enzymes in topic and ectopic endometrium, on the other hand, we have not found, so far, any studies that have evaluated the expression of these enzymes in granulosa cells of patients with endometriosis, whose anomalies could contribute to the impairment of folliculogenesis and of the acquisition of oocyte competence to permit fertilization and support embryo development.

The above data suggest a trend to a greater production of free radicals in endometriosis patients associated with a potential alteration of antioxidant capacity. This may contribute to oxidative stress which could be related to the pathogenesis and progression of endometriosis.

Another very interesting aspect of endometriosis is its enigmatic association with infertility, observed in 25 to 30% of women with this affection. Until now, little is known about the mechanisms involved in the pathogenesis of infertility, especially in minimal and mild endometriosis, where there is no significant alteration of pelvic anatomy.

New approaches to the treatment of infertility related to this disorder have included the increasingly more common application of ART. The introduction of *in vitro* fertilization (IVF) for the treatment of infertility secondary to endometriosis has become an important tool for the study of the potential effects of endometriosis on specific stages of the reproductive process, including folliculogenesis, fertilization, embryo development and implantation. Contradictory data have been reported for IVF outcomes in patients with endometriosis (García-Velasco & Arici, 1999; Garrido et al., 2000). This discrepancy seems to be multifactorial since IVF outcomes might be affected by different variables, such as ovulation induction protocol, patient selection criteria, laboratory procedures, and embryo transfer technique, among other factors.

As previously said, contradictory data have been reported for IVF outcomes in patients with endometriosis (Garrido et al., 2002; Garcia-Velasco & Arici, 1999; Kumbak et al., 2008; Fernando et al., 2008). Some studies suggest lower fertilization, implantation, and pregnancy rates in women with endometriosis (Barnhart et al., 2002; Al-Fadhli et al., 2006), possibly owing to impaired oocyte quality with consequent poor embryo quality, or to endometrial defects or defective interactions between the endometrium and the embryo (Kumbak et al., 2008, Brizek et al., 1995; Pellicer et al., 1995). Conflicting findings of some alterations in topic endometrium of endometriosis patients could explain, at least partially, the disturbance of the interaction between embryo and endometrium, generating anomalies in the implantation process (García-Velasco & Arici, 1999; Garrido et al., 2000). However, similar implantation rates in oocyte donation cycles have been recorded for women with endometriosis and control subjects, suggesting the crucial role of oocyte quality in impaired implantation processes (Pellicer et al., 1995; 2001; Díaz et al., 2000; Garrido et al., 2000; Katsoff et al., 2006). According to some authors, impaired oocyte quality would be responsible for compromising (Brizek et al., 1995) or completely blocking embryo development (Pellicer et al., 1995) in women with endometriosis, reinforcing the role of poor oocyte quality in the outcome of ART procedures in this group of patients.

Studies that intended to evaluate indirectly oocyte quality in patients with endometriosis analyzed multiple paracrine factors present in FF, such as interleukins, vascular endothelial growth factor (VEGF), and tumor necrosis factor (TNF), as well as granulosa cells apoptosis, leucocyte number and activity, among other indirect predictors of oocyte quality (Garrido et al., 2000, 2002). However, few studies have evaluated oocyte quality in patients with endometriosis by more objective morphological criteria.

Oocyte quality depends on factors related to the acquisition of nuclear and cytoplasmic competence. Although involving different processes, nuclear and cytoplasmic maturation are connected events that occur simultaneously in determined situations, although cytoplasmic molecular programming starts in the oocyte growth phase (Ferreira et al., 2009).

Nuclear competence depends on the anatomic and functional integrity of the meiotic spindle, a temporary and dynamic structure responsible for chromosomal segregation during meiosis (Wang & Keefe, 2002; Navarro et al., 2005). Meiotic anomalies might contribute to cell development failure by different paths, such as the inability of the oocyte to complete the maturation process in order to be fertilized, or the occurrence of variable errors of the meiotic maturation process that do not stop fertilization but might compromise embryo development pre or post implantation, as well as the future viability of the fetus (Armstrong, 2001; Chaube et al., 2005; Mansour et al., 2009). On the other hand, there is evidence that oxidative stress might promote meiotic anomalies and pre-implantation embryo development (Liu et al., 2003; Navarro et al., 2004, 2006; Agarwal et al., 2006; Mansour et al., 2009). Oxidative stress also seems to induce genomic and mitochondrial DNA damage (Aitken et al., 2001), which leads directly to reduced fertility (Guerin et al., 2001). Recently it was demonstrated that the peritoneal fluid of endometriosis patients promotes anomalies in oocyte cytoskeleton and increases embryo apoptosis, preventable by antioxidant supplementation (L-carnitine) in the culture medium, as shown in a study using mice as the experimental model (Mansour et al., 2009), suggesting that oxidative stress might be involved in the etiopathogenesis of poor oocyte quality in patients with this disease. In some recent studies, sperm incubated with peritoneal fluid of endometriosis patients showed increased DNA fragmentation and the extent of fragmentation increased according to endometriosis stage and infertility duration. Similarly, oocytes incubated with peritoneal fluid of endometriosis patients presented increased DNA damage and the extent of damage was proportional to the period of exposure. As expected, embryos incubated with peritoneal fluid also showed DNA fragmentation as indicated by an increase of apoptosis. The increase of DNA damage in spermatozoa, oocytes and embryos seems to be responsible for the numerous abortions and for fertilization and implantation failure among endometriosis patients (Mansour et al., 2009).

Our group was the first to assess the meiotic spindle and chromosome distribution of in vitro–matured (IVM) oocytes obtained from stimulated cycles of endometriosis patients and to compare them with a control group consisting of couples with male or tubal factors of infertility. We showed that, although IVM rates were similar for the two groups evaluated, a higher proportion of telophase I oocytes tended to occur in the endometriosis group. The number of oocytes was too low to detect statistically significant differences. However, this finding suggests a potential delay or impairment of meiosis I during IVM in the context of endometriosis. The mechanisms underlying this finding remain unclear. Recent studies demonstrated significant DNA damage and increased anomalies in the microtubules and chromosomes of oocytes incubated with PF from endometriosis patients (Mansour et al, 2009; Carbone et al., 2003), which were prevented by supplementation of the culture medium with the antioxidant L-carnitine, suggesting that impaired oocyte quality in endometriosis may be mediated by oxidative stress (Carbone et al., 2003). Although the data were obtained from frozen/thawed MII mouse oocytes and may not necessarily be extrapolated to human oocytes, they support our hypothesis that oxidative stress might be involved in the delay or impairment of meiosis I in oocytes of women with endometriosis (Barcelos et al., 2009), a possibility that requires more in-depth evaluation in future studies.

Unpublished data from our group suggest that this finding is also confirmed in in vivo matured oocytes of patients with moderate and severe endometriosis. However, we did not find well designed studies evaluating different pro and antioxidants markers in this group of patients, co-relating them with ART outcome as indirect predictors of oocyte quality.

If we have very little evidence correlating endometriosis and meiotic oocyte anomalies, data about the potential association between endometriosis and oocyte cytoplasmic maturation markers are even rarer. The gene expression of the antioxidant enzymatic system is one of the markers of oocyte cytoplasmic maturation, playing an important role by minimizing the hazardous effects of oxidative stress (Cetica et al., 2001). It has already been demonstrated that catalase, SOD and GPx are found in oocytes and COCs. GSH is one of the oocyte cytoplasmic maturation markers that have been intensely investigated. Some studies show that an adequate expansion of COCs, which is considered to be an oocyte maturation marker, is partially dependent on the intracellular concentration of GSH (Furnus et al., 1998). Intracellular GSH levels increase as the oocyte develops from germinal vesicle to metaphase II (Ali et al., 2003). After fertilization, the total amount of intracellular GSH correlates with spermatic chromatin decondensation, with consequent oocyte activation and also with the transformation of the sperm head to male pronucleus (De Matos & Furnus, 2000). However, no studies have evaluated the expression of this enzyme or of the entire GSH redox system in COCs of patients with infertility related to endometriosis. Matos et al. (2009) suggested a positive correlation between the SOD activity of COCs of infertile women submitted o ovarian stimulation for ART due to male factor and ART outcomes. In this same study an increase in SOD activity was observed in in vitro culture of COCs from infertile women with endometriosis. However, the authors analyzed the COCs of only six patients.

Some authors have associated minimal endometriosis with impaired steroidogenesis in granulosa cells, represented not only by a reduced baseline activity of aromatase, but also by a lower production of progesterone in non-stimulated and stimulated cycles (Harlow et al., 1996; Gomes et al., 2008). A functional failure of oocytes due to abnormal follicular function could be a result of this disease (Wardle et al., 1985). The antioxidants not only have an anti-apoptotic effect on preovulatory in vitro cultured follicles (Tsai-Turton & Luderer, 2006), but are also involved in the regulation of steroidogenic enzyme function dependent on cytochrome P450 (Verit et al., 2007). Some studies have suggested that ascorbic acid (Murray et al., 2001), as well as SOD (Lapolt & Hong, 1995) may have inhibitory effects on aromatase, an enzyme responsible for the conversion of androgens to estrogens, which could induce storage of androgens in the follicular fluid, leading to follicular atresia (Verit et al., 2007). As mentioned earlier, some recent data have demonstrated an increase of SOD activity in COCs (in vitro culture) of infertile women with endometriosis (Matos et al., 2009). Since no studies on endometriosis patients have evaluated antioxidant enzyme expression in luteinized granulosa cells and their correlation with steroidogenic enzymes dependent on cytochrome P450 expression, involved in ovarian steroidogenesis, our group has performed studies evaluating these possible associations.

7. Endometriosis, steroidogenesis and folliculogenesis

Some studies have shown an increase of luteinized unruptured follicle syndrome (LUF) and of the incidence of lutheal phase defects in women with endometriosis (Cheesman et al., 1983; Holtz et al., 1985; Saracoglu et al., 1985; Kaya & Oral, 1999). Other recent studies have shown a polymorphism of the progesterone gene and resistance to the action of progesterone in endometriosis tissues (Bulun et al., 2006; Van Kaam et al., 2007), supporting the hypothesis of impaired progesterone production and/or action in endometriosis (Bulun et al., 2006; Harlow et al., 1996). Some data show impaired steroidogenesis of granulosa cells associated with minimal endometriosis, represented not only by a reduction of basal aromatase activity, but also by a lower production of progesterone in stimulated as well as non-stimulated cycles (Harlow et al, 1996). Therefore, ovulatory dysfunction induced by impairment of ovarian steroid secretion as well as inadequate lutheal function might be important for the pathogenesis of infertility associated with endometriosis. A function defect in the oocyte due to abnormal follicle function might be the result of this ovulatory dysfunction (Wardle et al., 1985). Supporting this hypothesis, clinical studies involving IVF and some programs of oocyte donation have pointed out the importance of impaired oocyte quality in the pathogenesis of infertility associated with endometriosis (Pellicer et al., 1998; Garrido et al., 2002).

3β-Hydroxysteroide dehydrogenase/delta 5-delta 4-isomerase (3β-HSD) is an important enzyme associated with the biosynthesis of progesterone. Bar Ami (1994) evaluated the fertilization capacity related to the competence of granulosa cells and COCs to secrete progesterone. COCs from fertilized oocytes presented a 1.9 times higher progesterone level (p<0.001) on days 0-3 and a 1.6 times higher level (p<0.02) on days 3-5 of culture when compared to the levels in COCs of non-fertilized oocytes. Nevertheless, in COCs of fertilized oocytes, the activity of 3β-hydroxysteroid dehydrogenase was significantly higher after oocyte aspiration and also 3 to 5 days later compared to non-fertilized oocytes. These results suggest that, in stimulated cycles, in follicles that hold mature COCs there is a synchrony and correlation between competence to perform progesterone secretion by COCs as well as by granulosa cells and the potential of these oocytes to be fertilized. Such correlation suggests and supports the intimate relation of enzymatic activity of 3β-hydroxysteroid dehydrogenase and progesterone production with oocyte fertilization capacity, which may suggest the important role of this enzyme as coadjuvant in the acquisition of oocyte competence. The reduction of the gene expression and/or activity of this enzyme could lead to a lower production of progesterone and impairment of the luteal phase.

Aromatase is present in granulosa cells and actually plays a fundamental role in follicle maturation and in the establishment of oocyte quality (Erickson et al., 1989; Foldesi et al., 1998; Speroff & Fritz, 2005). But, if on the one hand we find evidence of increased aromatase expression in ectopic endometrium, on the other, there are poor and inconclusive data concerning the expression of this enzyme by luteinized granulosa cells, suggesting a lower activity of this enzyme, but with no confirmation of an associated lower gene expression.

It is known that oocyte quality results from a complex and synchronized process that lasts several months, from primordial follicle to pre-ovulatory follicle. This process starts in a gonadotropin-independent way and later becomes gonadotropin dependent. In this last phase, oocyte, granulosa cells and FSH interact synergically. Granulosa cell multiplication and the specific way they respond first to FSH and later to LH in order to produce intra-follicle steroids are crucial events in this process (Speroff & Fritz, 2005). We know that there are gap junctions between granulosa cells, which is evidence that there are molecular interactions between them and possibly with the oocyte itself, through signaling molecules such as growth and differentiation factor-9 (GDF-9) and bone morphogenetic protein-15 (BMP 15) (Albertini & Barrett, 2003; Combelles et al., 2004; Thomas & Vanderhyden, 2006; Hutt & Albertini, 2007). However, little information is available about the communication between granulosa cells and the oocyte.

Granulosa cells differentiate into mural and cumulus cells during folliculogenesis, a fact that has stimulated the study of their potential as mesenchymal stem cells. To date there are no studies comparing the gene expression of mural granulosa cells and COCs and, possibly, since they are cells with distinct function and differentiation, there might be genes with different patterns of expression. When they reach the pre-antral follicle stage, granulosa cells can synthetize all three types of steroids (androgens, progestagens and estrogens) (Speroff & Fritz, 2005). However, the proportions and timing of their production are crucial. It is known that FSH and also LH have hormonal receptors on granulosa cells and there is a synergism between these receptors and intra-follicle hormonal production to permit the development of a follicle that holds a mature oocyte (Costa et al., 2004; Speroff & Fritz, 2005; Silva et al., 2008). Androgens, for instance, are necessary at low concentrations at the very beginning of follicle development, as a substrate for estradiol production. According to the two cells theory, theca cells convert C21 components (cholesterol) to androgen, which is a substrate for the aromatase of granulosa cells that converts androgens (C19) to estrogens (C18). The transformation of an androgenic environment to an estrogenic one is crucial in order to produce an oocyte capable of ovulation (Speroff & Fritz, 2005). In granulosa cells, aromatase plays an essential role in folliculogenesis and in estradiol production and its expression increases with follicle development (Tetsuka &Hillier, 1997; Guet et al., 1999) under the influence of FSH (Speroff & Fritz, 2005). Therefore, aromatase is a crucial enzyme in granulosa cells which is responsible for the formation of an estrogenic follicle microenvironment, essential for development and maturation (Speroff & Fritz, 2005). Nevertheless, it is important to state that aromatase is the final point of the entire ovarian steroidogenic cascade and the only enzyme capable of converting androgens to estrogens. Therefore, if its activity is impaired, that specific follicle will have difficulty in acquiring a normal pre-ovulatory state.

Intra-follicle hormonal relations are essential for the success of the entire ovulatory process both in natural cycles and in cycles stimulated for ART. Regarding maturation, Costa et al. (2004) analyzed cycles stimulated with exogenous gonadotropins without using a GnRH analogue and found that the follicles that held mature oocytes presented an increase in the progesterone/testosterone (P/T) ratio), in the progesterone/estradiol (P/E2) ratio and in the estradiol/testosterone (E/T) ratio in follicular fluid when compared to immature oocytes, suggesting a decrease in C21 to C19 conversion, but not in aromatase activity. Silva et al. (2008) analyzed these same ratios in follicles of women submitted to stimulated cycles using a GnRH analogue and observed that the action of the analogue remained intact and its most important effect was a decrease in intra-follicle androgen, with higher rates of fertilization and maturation.

In vitro studies using granulosa cell culture of women with endometriosis submitted to ovarian hyperstimulated cycles showed that these cells present impaired aromatase activity. Harlow et al. (1996) investigated aromatase activity in patients with minimal and mild endometriosis using granulosa cell culture in which estrogen production was evaluated after adding testosterone to the culture medium. They found a decrease in aromatase activity in patients with endometriosis compared to control. Researchers from the same group (Cahill et al., 2003) using the same technique found a lower sensitivity to LH in granulosa cells of patients with endometriosis.

Abreu et al. (2006) found a reduction of estradiol production in *in vitro* luteinized mural granulosa cells of women with endometriosis, after 24 hours of cell culture. Under baseline conditions or when the culture medium was supplemented with a lower concentration of testosterone ($2 \times 10^{-6}M$), estradiol production was lower in the endometriosis group. However, when the concentration of testosterone (an aromatase precursor) added to the culture medium was increased ($2 \times 10^{-5}M$), there was no difference between the endometriosis and control groups concerning estradiol production. In another study performed by Abreu et al. (2009) no difference in aromatase gene expression (CYP19A1) was observed in luteinized mural cells of women with endometriosis and controls submitted to

ART. However, data obtained by the analysis of gene expression of mural granulosa cells of patients with endometriosis cannot be necessarily extrapolated to cumulus oophorus cells (COCs).

We found evidence that COCs might contribute to oocyte cytoplasmic maturation (Tanghe et al., 2002) through a net of gap junctions between COCs and between these and the oocyte (Furger et al., 1996). Nevertheless, the presence of COCs is important for fertilization to occur (Tanghe et al., 2002) because it attracts selected spermatozoa and promotes their capacitation and penetration. On the other hand, it should be emphasized that COCs protect the oocyte against apoptosis induced by oxidative stress (Tatemoto et al., 2000), which occurs when there is a large number of ROS compared to the anti-oxidants available. Some studies have suggested that analysis of gene expression of COCs might be used as an indirect predictor of oocyte quality and of the outcome of ART procedures, which could lead to distinct clinical applications (Hamamah et al., 2006; Assou et al., 2006, 2008; Hamel et al., 2008; Tesfaye et al., 2009; Haouzi & Hamamah, 2009).

In the female reproductive system, ROS and anti-oxidants play physiological roles during folliculogenesis, oocyte maturation, luteal regression and fertilization (Agarwal et al., 2006). For example, an increase in ROS production in granulosa cells (Jancar et al., 2007) and on oxidative damage to DNA marker (8-hydroxy-20-deoxyguanosine) levels in granulosa cells and COCs (Seino et al., 2002) was associated with lower fertilization, poor embryo quality and reduction of implantation rates. Nevertheless, oxidative stress also seems to be associated with the etiopathogenesis of reproduction, as is the case in endometriosis (Guerin et al., 2001; Van Langendonckt et al., 2002; Agarwal et al., 2003; Barcelos et al., 2008), idiopathic infertility and polycystic ovary syndrome (Gonzalez et al., 2006).

Considering this substantial involvement of ROS and oxidative stress in fertilization and reproduction modulation, it is accepted that anti-oxidant enzymes on COCs modulate oocyte maturation and might be related to specific conditions that limit the success of ART. Some studies have shown that superoxide dismutase (La Polt & Hong, 1995) might have inhibitory effects on aromatase, suggesting a potential correlation between gene expression of one of the major anti-oxidant enzymatic system and aromatase expression.

8. References

Abreu LG, Romão GS, Dos Reis RM, Ferriani RA, De Sá MF, De Moura MD. Reduced aromatase activity in granulosa cells of women with endometriosis undergoing assisted reproduction techniques. Gynecol Endocrinol. 2006 Aug;22(8):432-6.

Agarwal A, Gupta S, Sharma R. Role of oxidative stress in female reproduction. Reprod Biol Endocrinol. 2005; 3:28.

Agarwal A, Said TM, Bedaiwy MA, et al. Oxidative stress in an assisted reproductive techniques setting. Fertil Steril. 2006; 86(3):503-12.

Agarwal A, Saleh RA, Bedaiwy MA. Role of reactive oxygen species in the pathophysiology of human reproduction. Fertil Steril. 2003, 79(4):829-843.

Aitken RJ, Krausz C. Oxidative stress, DNA damage and the Y chromosome. Reproduction 2001;122:497–506.

Albertini DF, Barrett SL. Oocyte-somatic cell communication. Reproduction. 2003 61:49-54. 2003.

Al-Fadhli R, Kelly SM, Tulandi T, Tanr SL. Effects of different stages of endometriosis on the outcome of in vitro fertilization. J Obstet Gynaecol Can 2006;28:888-91.

Ali AA, Bilodeau JF, Sirard MA. Antioxidant requirements for bovine oocytes varies during in vitro maturation, fertilization and development. Theriogenology. 2003 Feb;59(3-4):939-49.

Alpay Z, Saed GM, Diamond MP. Female infertility and free radicals: potential role in adhesions and endometriosis. J Soc Gynecol Investig. 2006; 13(6):390-8.

Amaral VF, Bydlowski SP, Peranovich TC, Navarro PA, Subbiah MT, Ferriani RA. Lipid peroxidation in the peritoneal fluid of infertile women with peritoneal endometriosis. Eur J Obstet Gynecol Reprod Biol. 2005 Mar 1;119(1):72-5.

Andrade AZ, Rodrigues JK, Dib LA, Romão GS, Ferriani RA, Jordão Junior AA, Navarro PA. Serum markers of oxidative stress in infertile women with endometriosis. Rev Bras Ginecol Obstet. 2010 Jun;32(6):279-85.

Armstrong DT. Effects of maternal age on oocyte developmental competence. Theriogenology. 2001; 55(6):1303-22.

Assou S, Anahory T, Pantesco V, Carrour1 T, Pellestor F, Klein B, Reyftmann L, Dechaud H, De Vos J, Hamamah S. The human cumulus-oocyte complex gene-expression profile Hum Reprod. 2006 July ; 21(7): 1705–1719.

Assou S, Haouzi D, Mahmoud K, Aouacheria A, Guillemin Y, Pantesco V, Rème T, Dechaud H, De Vos J, Hamamah S. A non-invasive test for assessing embryo potential by gene expression profiles of human cumulus cells: a proof of concept study. Mol Hum Reprod. 2008 ;14(12):711-9.

Babior BM. Superoxide: a two-edged sword. Bras J Biol Res. 1997; 30(2): 141-55.

Bar-Ami S. Increasing progesterone secretion and 3 beta-hydroxysteroid dehydrogenase activity of human cumulus cells and granulosa-lutein cells concurrent with successful fertilization of the corresponding oocyte. J Steroid Biochem Mol Biol. 1994 Dec;51(5-6):299-305.

Barcelos ID, Vieira RC, Ferreira EM, Araújo MC, Martins W de P, Ferriani RA, Navarro PA. Meiotic abnormalities of oocytes from patients with endometriosis submitted to ovarian stimulation. Rev Bras Ginecol Obstet. 2008 Aug;30(8):413-9.

Barcelos ID, Vieira RC, Ferreira EM, Martins WP, Ferriani RA, Navarro PA. Comparative analysis of the spindle and chromosome configurations of in vitro-matured oocytes from patients with endometriosis and from control subjects: a pilot study. Fertil Steril. 2009 Nov;92(5):1749-52. Epub 2009 Jun 12.

Barnhart K, Dungsmoor-Su R, Coutifaris C. Effect of endometriosis on in vitro fertilization. Fertil Steril. 2002; 77(6): 148-55.

Bornoden W. Antioxidant nutrients and protection from free radicals. In: Kotsonis FN, Mackey M, Hjelle JJ (eds). Nutritional Toxicolgy. New York, Raven Press 1994; 19-48.

Brizek CL, Schlaff S, Pellegrini VA, Frank JB, Worrilow KC. Increased incidence of aberrant morphological phenotypes in human embryogenesis--an association with endometriosis. J Assist Reprod Genet 1995;12:106-12.

Bulun SE, Ping Yin YHC, Imir G, et al. Progesterone resistance in endometriosis: link to failure to metabolize estradiol. Mol Cell Endocrinol 2006;248:94–103.

Cahill DJ, Harlow CR, Wardle PG. Pre-ovulatory granulosa cells of infertile women with endometriosis are less sensitive to luteinizing hormone. Am J Reprod Immunol. 2003 Feb;49(2):66-9.

Calvin HI, Grosshans K, Blake EJ. Estimation and manipulation of glutathione levels in prepuberal mouse ovaries and ova: relevance to sperm nucleus transformation in the fertilized egg. Gamete Res 1986.

Campos Petean C, Ferriani RA, Dos Reis RM, Dias de Moura M, Jordao AA, Jr., Navarro PA. Lipid peroxidation and vitamin E in serum and follicular fluid of infertile women with peritoneal endometriosis submitted to controlled ovarian hyperstimulation: a pilot study. Fertil Steril 2008.

Carbone MC, Tatone C, Delle Monache S, Marci R, Caserta D, Colonna R et al. Antioxidant enzymatic defences in human follicular fluid: characterization and age-dependent changes. Mol Hum Reprod 2003;9:639-43.

Cetica PD, Pintos LN, Dalvit GC, Beconi MT. Antioxidant enzyme activity and oxidative stress in bovine oocyte in vitro maturation. IUBMB Life. 2001 Jan;51(1):57-64.

Chaube SK, Prasad PV, Thakur SC, et al. Hydrogen peroxide modulates meiotic cell cycle and induces morphological features characteristic of apoptosis in rat oocytes cultured in vitro. Apoptosis. 2005; 10(4):863–874.

Cheesman KL, Cheesman SD, Chatterton Jr RT, Cohen MR. Alterations in progesterone metabolism and luteal function in infertile women with endometriosis. Fertil Steril 1983;40(5):590–5.

Combelles CM, Carabatsos MJ, Kumar TR, Matzuk MM, Albertini DF. Hormonal control of somatic cell oocyte interactions during ovarian follicle development. Mol Reprod Dev. 2004 Nov;69(3):347-55.

Costa LO, Mendes MC, Ferriani RA, Moura MD, Reis RM, Silva de Sá MF. Estradiol and testosterone concentrations in follicular fluid as criteria to discriminate between mature and immature oocytes. Braz J Med Biol Res. 2004 Nov;37(11):1747-55. Epub 2004 Oct 26.

de Matos DG, Furnus CC, Moses DF. Glutathione synthesis during in vitro maturation of bovine oocytes: role of cumulus cells. Biol Reprod. 1997 Dec;57(6):1420-5.

de Matos DG, Furnus CC. The importance of having high glutathione (GSH) level after bovine in vitro maturation on embryo development effect of beta-mercaptoethanol, cysteine and cystine. Theriogenology. 2000 Feb;53(3):761-71.

De Santis L, Cino I, Rabellotti E, Calzi F, Persico P, Borini A et al. Polar body morphology and spindle imaging as predictors of oocyte quality. Reprod Biomed Online 2005;11:36-42.

Díaz I, Navarro J, Blasco L, et al. Impact of stage III-IV endometriosis on recipients of sibling oocytes: matched case-control study. Fertil Steril. 2000;74(1):31-4.

Erickson GF, Garzo VG, Magoffin DA. Insulin-like growth factor-I regulates aromatase activity in human granulosa and granulosa luteal cells. J Clin Endocrinol Metab. 1989 Oct;69(4):716-24.

Fernando S, Breheny S, Jaques AM, Halliday JL, Baker G, Healy D. Preterm birth, ovarian endometriomata, and assisted reproduction technologies. Fertil Steril 2008.

Ferreira EM, Vireque AA, Adona PR, Meirelles FV, Ferriani RA, Navarro PA. Cytoplasmic maturation of bovine oocytes: structural and biochemical modifications and acquisition of developmental competence. Theriogenology. 2009 Mar 15;71(5):836-48. Epub 2009 Jan 3. Review.

Földesi I, Breckwoldt M, Neulen J. Oestradiol production by luteinized human granulosa cells: evidence of the stimulatory action of recombinant human follicle stimulating hormone. Hum Reprod. 1998 Jun;13(6):1455-60.

Fujii J, Iuchi Y, Okada F. Fundamental roles of reactive oxygen species and protective mechanisms in the female reproductive system. Reprod Biol Endocrinol. 2005; 3:43.

Furger C, Cronier L, Poirot C, Pouchelet M. Human granulosa cells in culture exhibit functional cyclic AMP-regulated gap junctions. Mol Hum Reprod. 1996 Aug;2(8):541-8.

Furnus CC, de Matos DG, Moses DF. Cumulus expansion during in vitro maturation of bovine oocytes: relationship with intracellular glutathione level and its role on subsequent embryo development. Mol Reprod Dev. 1998 Sep;51(1):76-83

García-Velasco J, Arici A. Is endometrium or the oocyte/embryo affected in endometriosis? Hum Reprod. 1999; 14 (Suppl. 2):77-89.

Garrido N, Navarro J, Garcia-Velasco J, Remohi J, Pellice A, Simon C. The endometrium versus embryonic quality in endometriosis-related infertility. Hum Reprod Update 2002;8:95-103.

Garrido N, Navarro J, Remohi J, Simon C, Pellicer A. Follicular hormonal environment and embryo quality in women with endometriosis. Hum Reprod Update 2000;6:67-74.

Gomes FM, Navarro PA, de Abreu LG, Ferriani RA, dos Reis RM, de Moura MD. Effect of peritoneal fluid from patients with minimal/mild endometriosis on progesterone release by human granulosa-lutein cells obtained from infertile patients without endometriosis: a pilot study. Eur J Obstet Gynecol Reprod Biol. 2008;138(1):60-5.

González F, Rote NS, Minium J, Kirwan JP. Reactive oxygen species-induced oxidative stress in the development of insulin resistance and hyperandrogenism in polycystic ovary syndrome. J Clin Endocrinol Metab. 2006 Jan;91(1):336-40. Epub 2005 Oct 25.

Guérin P, El Mouatassim S, Ménézo Y. Oxidative stress and protection against reactive oxygen species in the pre-implantation embryo and its surroundings. Hum Reprod Update. 2001; 7(2):175-89.

Guet P, Royère D, Paris A, Lansac J, Driancourt MA. Aromatase activity of human granulosa cells in vitro: effects of gonadotrophins and follicular fluid. Hum Reprod. 1999 May;14(5):1182-9.

Gupta S, Agarwal A, Kraicir N, et al. Role of oxidative stress in endometriosis. Reprod Biomed Online. 2006; 13(1):126-34.

Halliwell B. Free radicals, antioxidants and human disease: curiosity, cause or consequence? Lancet. 1994; 344(8924):721-4.

Hamamah S, Matha V, Berthenet C, Anahory T, Loup V, Dechaud H, Hedon B, Fernandez A, Lamb N. Comparative protein expression profiling in human cumulus cells in relation to oocyte fertilization and ovarian stimulation protocol. Reprod Biomed Online. 2006;13(6):807-14.

Hamel M, Dufort I, Robert C, Gravel C, Leveille MC, Leader A, Sirard MA. Identification of differentially expressed markers in human follicular cells associated with competent oocytes. Hum Reprod. 2008;23(5):1118-27.

Hansen JC, Deguchi Y: Selenium and fertility in animals and man – a review. Acta Vet Scand 1996, 37:19-30.

Haouzi D, Hamamah S. Pertinence of Apoptosis Markers for the Improvement of In Vitro Fertilization (IVF). Curr Med Chem. 2009;16(15):1905-16.

Harlow CR, Cahill DJ, Maile LA, et al. Reduced preovulatory granulosa cell steroidogenesis in women with endometriosis. J Clin Endocrinol Metab 1996;81:426–9.

Ho YS, Magnenat JL, Bronson RT, Cao J, Gargano M, Sugawara M, Funk CD: Mice deficient in cellular glutathione peroxidase develop normally and show no increased sensitivity to hyperoxia. J Biol Chem 1997, 272:16644-16651.

Holtz G, Williamson HO, Mathur RS, Landgrebe SC, Moore EE. Luteinized unruptured follicle syndrome in mild endometriosis assessment with biochemical parameters. J Reprod Med 1985;30(9):643–5.

Hu Y, Betzendahl I, Cortvrindt R, Smitz J, Eichenlaub-Ritter U. Effects of low O2 and ageing on spindles and chromosomes in mouse oocytes from pre-antral follicle culture. Hum Reprod 2001;16:737-48.

Hutt KJ, Albertini DF. An oocentric view of folliculogenesis and embryogenesis. Reprod Biomed Online. 2007 Jun;14(6):758-64.

Jana SK, K NB, Chattopadhyay R, Chakravarty B, Chaudhury K. Upper control limit of reactive oxygen species in follicular fluid beyond which viable embryo formation is not favorable. Reprod Toxicol. 2010 Jul;29(4):447-51.

Jancar N, Kopitar AN, Ihan A, Virant Klun I, Bokal EV. Effect of apoptosis and reactive oxygen species production in human granulosa cells on oocyte fertilization and blastocyst development. J Assist Reprod Genet. 2007 Feb-Mar;24(2-3):91-7.

Jozwik M, Wolczynski S, Szamatowicz M. Oxidative stress markers in preovulatory follicular fluid in humans. Mol Hum Reprod 1999;5:409-13.

Katsoff B, Check JH, Davies E, Wilson C. Evaluation of the effect of endometriosis on oocyte quality and endometrial environment by comparison of donor and recipient outcomes following embryo transfer in a shared oocyte program. Clin Exp Obstet Gynecol. 2006; 33(4):201-2.

Kaya H, Oral B. Effect of ovarian involvement on the frequency of luteinized unruptured follicle in endometriosis. Gynecol Obstet Invest 1999;48(2):123–6.

Kim NH, Chung HM, Cha KY, Chung KS. Microtubule and microfilament organization in maturing human oocytes. Hum Reprod 1998;13:2217-22.

Kumbak B, Kahraman S, Karlikaya G, Lacin S, Guney A. In vitro fertilization in normoresponder patients with endometriomas: comparison with basal simple ovarian cysts. Gynecol Obstet Invest 2008;65:212-6.

LaPolt PS, Hong LS. Inhibitory effects of superoxide dismutase and cyclic guanosine 30,50-monophosphate on estrogen production in cultured rat granulosa cells. Endocrinology 1995;136:5533–9.

Liu L, Trimarchi JR, Navarro P, Blasco MA, Keefe DL. Oxidative stress contributes to arsenic-induced telomere attrition, chromosome instability, and apoptosis. J Biol Chem 2003;278:31998-2004.

Mandelbaum J, Anastasiou O, Levy R, Guerin JF, de Larouziere V, Antoine JM. Effects of cryopreservation on the meiotic spindle of human oocytes. Eur J Obstet Gynecol Reprod Biol 2004;113 Suppl 1:S17-23.

Mansour G, Abdelrazik H, Sharma RK, Radwan E, Falcone T, Agarwal A. L-carnitine supplementation reduces oocyte cytoskeleton damage and embryo apoptosis induced by incubation in peritoneal fluid from patients with endometriosis. Fertil Steril. 91(5 Suppl):2079-86, 2009

Matos L, Stevenson D, Gomes F, Silva-Carvalho JL, Almeida H. Superoxide dismutase expression in human cumulus oophorus cells Molecular Human Reproduction, Vol.15, No.7 pp. 411–419, 2009

Meister A. Selective modification of glutathione metabolism. Science 1983; 220:472-477.

Murphy AA, Santanam N, Parthasarathy S. Endometriosis: A disease of oxidative stress? Semin Reprod Endocrinol. 1998; 16(4):263-73.

Murray AA, Molinek MD, Baker SJ, Kojima FN, Smith MF, Hillier SG, et al. Role of ascorbic acid in promoting follicle integrity and survival in intact mouse ovarian follicles in vitro. Reproduction 2001;121:89–96.

Navarro PA, Liu L, Ferriani RA, Keefe DL. Arsenite induces aberrations in meiosis that can be prevented by coadministration of N-acetylcysteine in mice. Fertil Steril 2006;85 Suppl 1:1187-94.

Navarro PA, Liu L, Keefe DL. In vivo effects of arsenite on meiosis, preimplantation development, and apoptosis in the mouse. Biol Reprod. 2004; 70(4):980-5.

Navarro PA, Liu L, Trimarchi JR, et al. Noninvasive imaging of spindle dynamics during mammalian oocyte activation. Fertil Steril. 2005; 83(Suppl 1):1197-205.

Paszkowski T, Traub AI, Robinson SY, McMaster D: Selenium dependent glutathione peroxidase activity in human follicular fluid. Clin Chim Acta 1995, 236:173-180).

Pellicer A, Navarro J, Bosch E, Garrido N, Garcia-Velasco JA, Remohí J, Simón C. Endometrial quality in infertile women with endometriosis. Ann N Y Acad Sci. 2001 Sep;943:122-30. Review.

Pellicer A, Oliveira N, Ruiz A, Remohi J, Simon C. Exploring the mechanism(s) of endometriosis-related infertility: an analysis of embryo development and implantation in assisted reproduction. Hum Reprod 1995;10 Suppl 2:91-7.

Pellicer A, Valbuena D, Bauset C, et al. The follicular environment in stimulated cycles of women with endometriosis: esteroid levels and embryo quality. Fertil Steril 1998;69:1135–41.

Perreault SD, Barbee RR, Slott VI. Importance of glutathione in the acquisition and maintenance of sperm nuclear decondensing activity in maturing hamster oocytes. . Dev Biol. 1988 Jan;125(1):181-6.

Perreault SD, Wolff RA, Zirkin BR. The role of disulfide bond reduction during mammalian sperm nuclear decondensation in vivo. Dev Biol. 1984 Jan;101(1):160-7.

Revised American Society for Reproductive Medicine classification of endometriosis: 1996. Fertil Steril. 1997 May;67(5):817-21. [No authors listed]

Sabatini L, Wilson C, Lower A, Al-Shawaf T, Grudzinskas JG Superoxide dismutase activity in human follicular fluid after controlled ovarian hyperstimulation in women undergoing in vitro fertilization. Fertil Steril 1999, 72:1027-1034.].

Saracoglu OF, Aksel S, Yeoman RR,Wiebe RH. Endometrial estradiol and progesterone receptors in patients with luteal phase defects and endometriosis. Fertil Steril 1985;43(6):851–5.

Seino T, Saito H, Kaneko T, Takahashi T, Kawachiya S, Kurachi H. Eight-hydroxy-2'-deoxyguanosine in granulosa cells is correlated with the quality of oocytes and embryos in an in vitro fertilization-embryo transfer program. Fertil Steril. 2002 Jun;77(6):1184-90.

Silva AL, Abreu LG, Rosa-e-Silva AC, Ferriani RA, Silva-de-Sá MF. Leuprolide acetate reduces both in vivo and in vitro ovarian steroidogenesis in infertile women undergoing assisted reproduction. Steroids. 2008 Dec 22;73(14):1475-84. Epub 2008 Aug 26.

Speroff L, Fritz MA. Regulation of the Menstrual Cycle. In: Speroff L & Fritz MA. Clinical Gynecologic Endocrinology and Infertility. 7 ed. Baltimore: Lippincott Williams & Wilkins p. 187-231: 2005.

Szczepanska M, Kozlik J, Skrzypczak J, et al. Oxidative stress may be a piece in the endometriosis puzzle. Fertil Steril. 2003; 79(6):1288-93.

Tanghe S, Van Soom A, Nauwynck H, Coryn M, de Kruif A. Minireview: Functions of the cumulus oophorus during oocyte maturation, ovulation, and fertilization. Mol Reprod Dev. 2002 Mar;61(3):414-24.

Tatemoto H, Sakurai N, Muto N. Protection of porcine oocytes against apoptotic cell death caused by oxidative stress during In vitro maturation: role of cumulus cells. Biol Reprod. 2000 Sep;63(3):805-10.

Tesfaye D, Ghanem N, Carter F, Fair T, Sirard MA, Hoelker M, Schellander K, Lonergan P Gene expression profile of cumulus cells derived from cumulus-oocyte complexes matured either in vivo or in vitro. Reprod Fertil Dev. 2009;21(3):451-61.

Tetsuka M, Hillier SG. Differential regulation of aromatase and androgen receptor in granulosa cells. J Steroid Biochem Mol Biol. 1997 Apr;61(3-6):233-9.

Thomas FH, Vanderhyden BC. Oocyte-granulosa cell interactions during mouse follicular development: regulation of kit ligand expression and its role in oocyte growth. Reprod Biol Endocrinol. 2006 Apr 12;4:19.

Tsai-Turton M, Luderer U. Opposing effects of glutathione depletion and follicle-stimulating hormone on reactive oxygen species and apoptosis in cultured preovulatory rat follicles. Endocrinology 2006;147:1224–36.

Van Blerkom J, Davis P. Differential effects of repeated ovarian stimulation on cytoplasmic and spindle organization in metaphase II mouse oocytes matured in vivo and in vitro. Hum Reprod 2001;16:757-64.

Van Kaam KJ, Romano A, Schouten JP, Dunselman GA, Groothuis PG. Progesterone receptor polymorphism +331G/A is associated with a decreased risk of deep infiltrating endometriosis. Hum Reprod 2007;22(1):129–35.

Van Langendonckt A, Casanas-Roux F, Donnez J. Oxidative stress and peritoneal endometriosis. Fertil Steril. 2002; 77(5):861-70.

Verit FF, Erel O, Kocyigit A, Association of increased total antioxidant capacity and anovulation in nonobese infertile patients with clomiphene citrate–resistant polycystic

Volarcik K, Sheean L, Goldfarb J, Woods L, Abdul-Karim FW, Hunt P. The meiotic competence of in-vitro matured human oocytes is influenced by donor age: evidence that folliculogenesis is compromised in the reproductively aged ovary. Hum Reprod 1998;13:154-60.

Wang WH, Keefe DL. Prediction of chromosome misalignment among in vitro matured human oocytes by spindle imaging with the PolScope. Fertil Steril 2002;78:1077-81.

Wardle PG, Mitchell JD, McLaughlin EA, Ray BD, McDermott A, Hull MG. Endometriosis and ovulatory disorder: reduced fertilization in vitro compared with tubal and unexplained infertility. Lancet 1985; 2(8449):236-9.

Yoshida M, Ishigaki K, Pursel VG. Effect of maturation media on male pronucleus formation in pig oocytes matured in vitro. Mol Reprod Dev 1992; 31:68-71.

Yoshida M. Role of glutathione in the maturation and fertilization ofpig oocytes in vitro. Mol Reprod Dev 1993; 35:76-81.

7

Embryo Quality and Pregnancy Outcome in Infertile Patients with Endometriosis

Veljko Vlaisavljević, Marko Došen and Borut Kovačič
Department of Reproductive Medicine and Gynecologic Endocrinology,
Clinics for Gynecology and Perinatology, University Clinical Center Maribor,
Slovenia

1. Introduction

Investigation of one complex pathological condition is definitively a challenging task, but trying to find the connection(s) between two is even more difficult. This is very true in the case of infertility and endometriosis. Both conditions have numerous symptoms, very diverse clinical pictures and multifactorial etiologies. The first step toward understanding the connection between the two is to prove the correlation between them. The next task is to try to understand the mechanisms by which they affect each other, which involves examination and comparison of numerous variables specific for each condition. The results are still the subject of many controversies.

1.1 Endometriosis and infertility

At present, there is little debate that endometriosis and infertility are actually associated. For example, early retrospective studies (Hasson, 1976; Drake & Grunet, 1980; Strathy et al., 1982) and one more recent prospective study (Mahmood & Templeton, 1991) performed in women who underwent laparoscopy (for various reasons) showed that endometriotic lesions were significantly more frequent in women who were treated for infertility than in those who requested laparoscopy for tubal sterilization. Prevalence of endometriosis in infertile women ranged from 21 - 48% which was in clear contrast to the prevalence of 1.3 - 5% in fertile women (Hasson, 1976; Drake & Grunet, 1980; Strathy et al., 1982). Another line of evidence of the existence of a link between endometriosis and infertility came from studies in women who underwent donor insemination because of severe male infertility. In these studies, women with endometriosis had significantly fewer conceptions per procedure than women without this condition (Hammond et al., 1986; Yeh & Seibel, 1987). In studies where peritoneal endometriosis was induced in rabbits (Schenken & Asch, 1980), primates (Schenken et al., 1984) and rodents (Vernon & Wilson 1985; Barragan et al., 1992) it was clearly demonstrated that endometriosis was strongly associated with infertility regardless of localization and/or extension of the lesions.

While it is relatively easy to document the link between the two conditions, defining precise pathophysiologic mechanisms and proving a causal relationship between endometriosis and infertility is much more difficult.

In severe cases of endometriosis, the seriously distorted anatomy of pelvic organs is the obvious cause of impaired fertility. In the absence of pelvic adhesions and scarring, when only mild to moderate endometriotic lesions are present, finding the cause and the consequence is anything but an easy task. Many confounding factors make these studies both controversial and difficult to interpret. One of the main problems is the choice of the appropriate control group. The common practice has been to choose women with tubal factor infertility or those with unexplained infertility as controls. The problem with this choice is our inability to identify women with inherently reduced potential for conception (fertilization and implantation) and to exclude them from the control group. Also, the common practice is to make observations on the patients with endometriosis who are treated by one of the techniques of assisted reproductive technologies (ART). This practice is problematic because the use of ART creates a non-physiologic environment and many subtle but important *in vivo* effects of endometriosis on the process of conception may be hidden in *in vitro* conditions.

Hypotheses on mechanisms by which mild to moderate endometriosis could impair fertility potential are numerous and will be mentioned here only briefly. One group of investigators tested hypotheses that endocrine abnormalities in women with mild and moderate endometriosis might be the cause of reduced fertility. As was already conveniently summarized in the literature (Garrido et al., 2000; Hunter et al., 2004), proposed mechanisms were hypersecretion of prolactin in patients with endometriosis (Muse et al., 1982), impaired folliculogenesis (Tummon et al., 1988), altered ovulation (Dmowski et al., 1986) and luteal phase defects (Grant, 1966). The other line of investigation was directed towards immune dysfunctions as potential causes of infertility in patients with endometriosis. Proposed mechanisms were chronic inflammatory reaction and altered immune responses induced by endometriosis (Harada et al., 2001), including increased production of cytokines and other soluble immunomodulators in the peritoneal fluid. These altered immune responses could further affect motility and velocity of the sperm, lead to sperm phagocytosis (Soldati et al., 1989), accelerate ovum transport (Croxato et al., 1978), impair the process of fertilization (Mahadevan et al., 1983), display direct embryo toxicity (Damewood et al., 1990) or adversely affect the process of implantation (Yovich et al., 1985; Matson & Yovich, 1986). Unfortunately, results of these studies were usually contradicting and no definitive conclusion could be made so far. It is likely that there is more than one answer to this complex problem.

2. Endometriosis and embryo quality

Among investigators who reported poorer results of IVF-ET outcome in patients with endometriosis, there is a general agreement on few final consequences in contrast to numerous possible pathophysiologic mechanisms leading to it.

These include:

1. Impairment of the quality of oocytes (resulting in lower fertilization rates) and/or
2. Decrease in the implantation capacity of embryos (Pellicer et al., 2001).

An indirect marker of oocyte quality and a possible predictor of embryo's implantation capacity is the quality of the developing embryo. As such, this parameter could be used for assessment of the effects of endometriosis on fertility.

2.1 Measures of embryo quality

Quality of the embryo may be described using many direct and indirect measures. For example, parameters which could be used for indirect assessment of embryo quality are number of embryos on Day 2, total number of blastocysts, number of frozen blastocysts, but also the implantation rate and early pregnancy loss rate. The only direct measure of embryo quality is embryo quality score based on morphological characteristics of a developing embryo. However, this parameter is quite difficult to use in practice. One reason for this difficulty is the absence of uniformity of scoring systems used by different laboratories. Another is a consequence of two facts: (1) quality score is a categorical variable and (2) it is (still) a common practice to transfer more than one embryo (blastocyst) at a time. In other words, if two or more embryos of different qualities have been transferred, it is not possible to calculate "the mean embryo quality score" or to determine exactly which one of transferred embryos has eventually implanted.

Researchers who would come across this issue tried to overcome it in various ways. The simplest was to exclude from the study those patients in whom embryos with different quality scores were transferred (La Sala et al., 2005). The main drawback of this approach was a significant reduction of observed cycles, i.e. of the sample size. Also, this tactic prevented incorporation of some other important variables (namely the number of transferred embryos) in the final analysis. On the other hand, some of the authors (Lambers et al, 2007) used a cumulative embryo score, previously introduced by Steer (Steer et al., 1992). Cumulative embryo score was defined as an additive parameter (i.e. following the transfer of two embryos with scores of 1 and 3, the total score of embryos transferred was 4). Other investigators (Winter et al., 2002) assessed embryo quality with relation to the number of embryos transferred and the possibility of elective transfer. According to this system, embryos were scored 1 in the case of an elective transfer of one or two embryos (highest score); elective transfer of 3 embryos yielded a score of 2; if two or three embryos had been transferred non-electively, the score was 3, and if only a single embryo was transferred non-electively, it was scored 4 (worst score).

In our research, we adopted yet another approach. If multiple embryos of different quality were transferred, we assumed that (1) implanting embryo was the best quality embryo (the so-called leading embryo) and (2) the leading embryo determined embryo quality score of the entire group of transferred embryos. The first assumption was well documented in the literature (Hourvitz et al., 2006) and the second one was additionally tested in our sample.

2.2 Relevant studies encompassing the measures of embryo quality

Despite the fact that important hypothesis blames defective early embryo development for poorer IVF-ET outcome in patients with endometriosis, relatively few studies have analyzed the association between quality of transferred embryo(s) and endometriosis. We will briefly present several important studies on the subject.

A group of Spanish investigators conducted three separate retrospective analyses of the success of their IVF-ET and oocyte donation program in patients and donors with and without endometriosis (Pellicer at al., 1995). In the segment of the study on early embryonic development, which was performed on 36 women with endometriosis and on 34 with tubal infertility used as a control group, they explored the embryos grown in vitro for 72 hours before embryo transfer. Embryo quality assessment system included the number of blastomeres and the degree of fragmentation after 48 and 72 hours in culture. If embryos presented only one or two blastomeres 72 hours after oocyte retrieval, it was considered that an embryo arrest had occurred. After 72 hours in culture, there was a significant decrease in the number of blastomeres in endometriosis compared to tubal infertility patients (5.4 ± 0.1 versus 6.1 ± 0.3 blastomeres, respectively, p<0.04) and a significant increase in the percentage of arrested embryos (57.4 ± 2.3 in patients with endometriosis versus 45.2 ± 5.8 in control group, p<0.05). In order to control for the influence of semen parameter on embryo quality, researchers further subdivided groups of patients taking into account the quality of semen. If abnormal semen was used for in vitro fertilization, higher degree of embryonic arrest was observed in comparison to the group with normal semen parameters (55.6 ± 6.4 vs. 20.3 ± 7.9 (p<0.01), respectively, in the group with tubal infertility; 61.8 ± 2.6 vs. 47.5 ± 2.8 (p<0.003), respectively, in the group with endometriosis). Also, if the semen used had normal characteristics, significantly more arrested embryos were noted in patients with endometriosis compared to patients with tubal infertility (p<0.001). Further insight into the problem was attained when the same researchers analyzed pregnancy outcome of oocyte donation with regards to the origin of donated oocytes. This segment of the research incorporated a total of 178 embryo transfers in 141 women. If oocytes were donated by donors without endometriosis, implantation and ongoing pregnancy rates were comparable in both recipients with and those without endometriosis. If oocytes were collected from donors with endometriosis, significantly lower implantation rates were reported in recipients (p<0.05). The authors of this study concluded that infertility in patients with endometriosis may be related to oocyte alterations which result in embryos of lower quality and reduced implantation ability, although the impact of hostile (anti-implantatory) environment on embryos of normal developmental potential cannot be ruled out.

Another study which reported negative impact of endometriosis on embryo quality was the prospective case control study in which researchers included 37 patients with "true" endometriomas and 56 patients without any complex ovarian cysts as controls (Yanushpolsky et al., 1998). All endometriomas were larger than 1 cm in diameter and would be classified as stage III endometriosis according to The ASRM-revised classification of endometriosis (The American Fertility Society, 1985). Only patients with complex "chocolate" cysts in which CA 125 levels in cyst fluid were >100.000 U/ml ("true" endometriomas) were included in the study. Embryo quality was expressed as the number of embryos reaching at least four-cell stage on the second day after oocyte retrieval. Quality of the embryos in the group of patients with endometriomas was significantly reduced compared to controls (p=0.09). Also, in patients with endometriomas, significantly fewer oocytes were retrieved (p=0.06) and early pregnancy loss rate (biochemical pregnancies and early clinical spontaneous miscarriages combined) was significantly higher (p=0.04). Interestingly, fertilization rate and implantation rate were not significantly different between the studied groups.

A group of Norwegian investigators also confirmed detrimental effect of endometriosis on embryo quality (Tanbo, 1995). They analyzed 215 women (385 cycles) whose main indication for IVF-ET was unexplained infertility (ovulatory women, with patent tubes and normal uterine cavity, normal laparoscopy and normal sperm characteristics), 143 women (285 cycles) with endometriosis as the only indication and 180 women (353 cycles) with tubal infertility (control group). Cleavage rate and failure of cleavage were used as criteria of embryo quality. Significantly lower cleavage rates were observed in both unexplained infertility and endometriosis groups compared with the tubal infertility group. Total failure of cleavage was 19.2% in unexplained infertility, 14.3% in endometriosis and 3.6% in tubal infertility group (p<0.0001). Since there were no differences in sperm characteristics between the groups, the authors speculated that lower cleavage rates could be a consequence of inferior oocyte quality in unexplained infertility and endometriosis group.

In an interesting study of authors from U.S.A. a total of 235 preimplantation embryos were retrospectively analyzed (Brizek et al., 1995). These embryos were obtained from 56 IVF-ET cycles performed in 30 women. Sixteen patients had endometriosis as the main indication for the procedure and the remaining 14 were controls without endometriosis who were chosen randomly from other diagnosis categories. The incidence of specific phenotypes ranging from normal 2PN zygote to different types of abnormal embryos was then recorded on days 1 and 2 following fertilization. An increased incidence of aberrant development of embryos derived from women with endometriosis was demonstrated. There were three abnormal phenotypes on day 1 and two abnormal phenotypes on day 2 which were significantly more prevalent in patients with endometriosis. However, there was no statistical difference in the number of normal embryos in patients with endometriosis compared to controls on day 1 or day 2. Despite the fact that the effect of endometriosis was observed in the developmental dynamics of the fertilized ovum, no gross endometriosis-specific morphological changes in oocytes recovered from endometriosis group could be seen.

In contrast to previously cited observations, several other studies failed to show negative influence of endometriosis on the parameters of embryo quality. A group of authors from the U.S.A. conducted a retrospective analysis of 284 IVF-ET cycles from patients with a sole diagnosis of endometriosis, or tubal factor, or unexplained infertility (Arici et al., 1996). All of the patients had laparoscopy prior to the IVF procedure. The criteria for the diagnosis of unexplained infertility were confirmed ovulatory cycles, normal tubal patency on hysterosalpingography, normal sperm analyses. The severity of endometriosis was graded as defined by the Revised American Fertility Society classification (The American Fertility Society, 1985) and patients were further divided into two subgroups as minimal to mild (stages I and II) and moderate to severe (stages III and IV). Quality of embryos was assessed on the day of the transfer in line with the system used by the authors' center according to their morphology as observed under the inverted microscope (morphological grades I to V). In the final analysis, the researchers used "the average embryo quality score" for the given subgroup of patients, which was probably calculated as the arithmetical average of all embryo quality scores expressed as grades I to V. No statistically significant difference in "average embryo score" among subgroups were noted (1.8 ± 0.5 in the minimal to mild endometriosis group vs. 2.0 ± 0.6 in the moderate to severe endometriosis group vs. 1.9 ± 0.5 in the tubal infertility group vs. 1.8 ± 0.6 in the unexplained infertility group; p>0.05). Surprisingly, when the data were analyzed according to the stage of endometriosis, in the group with moderate to severe endometriosis (stages III and IV) a significantly higher fertilization rate was observed compared to the group with minimal to mild endometriosis (stages I and II) (78.4% vs. 66.8%, respectively; p=0.001). However, implantation rates were low and not significantly different between these subgroups (5.5% in the group with moderate to severe endometriosis vs. 2.8% in the group with minimal to mild endometriosis, p=0.46).

Another study which failed to show negative impact of endometriosis on embryo quality was conducted by Swedish researchers (Bergendal et al., 1998). The analysis included a total of 65 IVF-ET cycles in 48 patients with endometriosis as the only apparent cause of infertility and 98 cycles in 98 patients in whom tubal factor was the only apparent cause of infertility (controls). The embryos were graded according to criteria set by the authors' center (morphology and cleavage stage) with embryo quality scores raging from 1 to 3, with 3 being the best score. The average score of the whole subgroup (defined as arithmetical average of all scores) was used in the final analysis. Despite the fact that fertilization rate was significantly higher in patients with tubal infertility compared to patients with endometriosis (78.3 ± 18.3% vs. 60.1 ± 31.7%, respectively; p=0.00001), no difference was noted in cleavage rates (87.9 ± 19.1% in the tubal factor group vs. 85.2 ± 22.1% in the endometriosis group; p=0.43) or morphological score of embryo for ET (2.5 ±0.39 in the tubal infertility group vs. 2.4 ± 0.4 in the endometriosis group; p=0.45).

In yet another study which reported results on the impact of endometriosis on embryo quality (Dmowski et al., 1995), a retrospective analysis of 237 consecutive IVF-ET cycles in patients with and without endometriosis was conducted. In the group without endometriosis, indications for IVF-ET were tubal disease, pelvic adhesions, male factor, unexplained infertility, ovarian dysfunction ant other factors. In this study, the number of oocytes cleaved was taken as the indirect measure of embryo quality. The authors reported there was no difference between groups in the number of fertilized and cleaved oocytes, but no exact numerical values for these variables were included in the published report. The lack of properly defined control group (endometriosis vs. all other indications) and the absence of further details on development of transferred embryos warrant caution for interpretation, at least in the segment of the study pertaining to embryo quality.

2.3 Our study

We conducted a retrospective clinical study which encompassed 346 stimulated IVF or ICSI cycles with the transfer of one or two blastocysts performed at the Department of Reproductive Medicine and Gynecological Endocrinology at the University Medical Centre of Maribor, Slovenia.

The primary objective of our study was to examine possible differences in direct and indirect indicators of embryo quality between women with endometriosis as the only indication for the treatment and an adequate control group of women with tubal factor only. Possible differences in various other outcomes of IVF-ET cycles between these two groups were also analyzed. The secondary goal was to examine the influence of embryo quality on various outcomes of IVF-ET cycles against all other important variables as controls in the group of women with endometriosis.

2.3.1 Materils and methods

Data used in this analysis were received from the centre's database on couples treated for infertility from 2003 to 2010. If there any data for any variable was missing from the database, the patient's documentation (paper records) was checked. If it was still impossible to find the missing data, the patient was excluded from further analysis. Patients included were under 43 years of age and prior to entering an IVF/ICSI treatment, underwent all tests prescribed by the protocol for clinical examination of infertile couples.

The observed cycles were divided into two groups: 173 cycles were performed in patients with endometriosis as the only indication for treatment and 173 cycles in women with tubal factor infertility (control group). The patients from tubal factor group were individually matched with women with endometriosis by age group (<30, 30-34, 35-39, >39 years), number of retrieved oocytes (<5, 5 or more) and number of transferred embryos (1, 2 or 3).

Patients were most frequently stimulated according to the protocol involving gonadotrophin-releasing hormone agonists (GnRH-a) (almost exclusively using the long protocol). In the few remaining patients, the protocol with gonadotrophin-releasing hormone antagonists (GnRH-ant) was applied. GnRH agonists used were triptorelin (Diphereline®, Ipsen Pharma Biotech, France), gosereline (Zoladex®, Zeneca Pharmaceuticals, England) or busereline (Suprefact®, Sanofi Aventis, France). Cetrorelix (3 mg) (Cetrotide®, Merck Serono, Switzerland) was used as a GnRH antagonist. Follicle growth was predominantly stimulated by recombinant FSH (Gonal F®, Merck Serono, Switzerland), while human menopausal gonadotrophin (HMG) (Menopur ®, Ferring Pharmaceuticals, Switzerland) was used occasionally. On the day when at least two follicles reached an average diameter of 18 mm, final maturation of the oocyte was stimulated by the urinary human HCG (Profasi®, Merck Serono, Switzerland, using a dose of 10,000 IU) or human recombinant HCG (Ovitrelle®, Merck Serono, Switzerland, 250 mg dose). A detailed description of the laboratory procedures can be found elsewhere (Kovacic et al., 2009). Approximately 36 hours (36 ± 1) following the administration of HCG, oocytes were recovered by ultrasound-guided trans-vaginal follicle aspiration. Fertilization was performed through IVF or ICSI. Medicult® media (MediCult, Denmark) were used for oocyte culturing. Pursuant to the protocol of our centre, only one or maximally two blastocysts were transferred on the fifth, exceptionally on the fourth day following follicle aspiration. Labotec® catheter (Labotec, Germany) was used for blastocyst transfer. In line with the legislation in force at the time of the study, the couple was allowed to decide on the number of embryos to be transferred. Embryos were transferred only after both partners signed the official consent form for the transfer of embryos. A day after the follicle aspiration, all patients started receiving didrogesterone (30 mg/day) (Dabroston®, Belupo, Croatia) or micronized progesterone (600 mg/day) (Utrogestan®, Laboratories Besins International, France) for luteal support.

Quality of transferred blastocysts was evaluated by a blastocyst classification system based on morphological criteria, developed by our centre (Kovacic et al., 2004). This classification is a modification of the earlier, well established blastocyst evaluation system (Gardner & Schoolcraft, 1999). The classification used in our laboratory takes into consideration four parameters: blastocoel expansion, inner cellular mass (ICM) form, morphology and cohesion of the trophoectoderm (TE) as well as the degree of embryo fragmentation. There are 8 grades of quality of blastocysts (B1 to B8) in this system, with B1 being the best quality score and B8 the worst. The data on blastocyst quality expressed in this way had to be transformed before entering the statistical model. The transformation was performed in two steps. First, the blastocysts from B1 category were designated as optimal quality blastocysts, while those in categories B2–B8 were classified as being of suboptimal (non-optimal) quality. In the second step, in cases where blastocysts of different quality were transferred, the subgroup with blastocysts of different quality was merged with the subgroup in which all transferred blastocysts were of optimal quality. In this way, for the final statistical analyses we had a subgroup with blastocysts of suboptimal quality only and a subgroup with at least one blastocyst of optimal quality. All other possibilities for regrouping were also tested, but it was concluded that the chosen transformation of data showed the best fit with this model. This conclusion was expected, because it was in line with the assumption that in those cases in which multiple embryos of different quality were transferred and only one of implanted, the higher quality embryo (so-called leading embryo) had the highest probability of implantation.

In our analysis we made a distinction between premenstrual pregnancy loss (loss of conceptus prior to the first measurement of βhCG level 14 days after ovulation or embryo transfer), biochemical pregnancy (loss of conceptus after the first measurement of βhCG level but before the ultrasound (US) confirmation of implantation) and early clinical miscarriage (pregnancy loss after US confirmation of viable pregnancy but before the beginning of the second trimester) (Došen et al., 2011). Biochemical pregnancies and early clinical miscarriages are commonly identified together as early pregnancy losses (EPL).

Basic demographic and clinical characteristics are presented as mean ± standard deviation (SD) or median with 1st and 3rd quartile and analyzed by independent-samples t-test if normally distributed or by Mann-Whitney test if skewed. Categorical data are expressed as proportions and analyzed by chi-squared test. The results are presented as odds ratios and their 95% confidence intervals (CI). P value of under 0.05 was considered to be statistically significant. Statistical analysis was performed using STATISTICA® software, version 8.0 (StatSoft Inc., OK, USA).

2.3.2 Results

2.3.2.1 Differences in embryo quality indicators and other parameters between the groups

Average age of the patients was 32 years (in the group of women with endometriosis 32.6 ± 3.5, the youngest patient was 25 and the oldest 42 years old; in the group with tubal infertility 32.5 ± 3.9, the youngest patient was 22 and the oldest 43 years old).

Analysis of differences in quality score of transferred blastocysts between patients with endometriosis and tubal factor infertility showed marginal statistical significance, if all the scores (B1-B8) were analyzed together (chi-square=14.03, p=0.051). Further analysis was undertaken to identify the subgroups of the same blastocyst quality score in which possible significant difference was present. The results are presented in Table 1.

Blastocyst quality score	Endometriosis group (N=173)	Tubal factor group (N=173)	P value
B1	195 (24.8)	201 (25.2)	0.873
B2	54 (6.9)	70 (8.8)	0.161
B3	106 (13.5)	114 (14.3)	0.653
B4	85 (10.8)	71 (8.9)	0.198
B5	47 (6.0)	46 (5.8)	0.851
B6	105 (13.4)	140 (17.5)	0.022
B7	41 (5.2)	25 (3.1)	0.038
B8	153 (19.5)	132 (16.5)	0.127
Total	786 (100.0)	799 (100.0)	

Table 1. Comparison of embryo quality scores between the studied groups

Since a significant difference was present only in the subgroups of transferred blastocysts of very low quality (scores B6 and B7), this finding doesn't provide any further insight into the problem.

Analysis of indirect embryo quality indicators showed no statistically significant differences between the groups. The results are presented in Table 2.

Variable[a]	Endometriosis group (N=173)	Tubal factor group (N=173)	P value
No. of embryos on Day 2	7.5 ± 0.30	7.5 ± 0.29	0.890
No. of blastocysts	3.7 ± 0.21	4.0 ± 0.20	0.317
No. of frozen blastocysts	2.0 ± 0.18	2.4 ± 0.20	0.210

[a] Data are expressed as mean ± standard error.

Table 2. Comparison of indirect indicators of embryo quality between the studied groups.

Analysis of outcomes of IVF-ET cycles also failed to show any statistically significant differences between the groups. Results are presented in Table 3.

The outcome	Endometriosis group (N=173)	Tubal factor group (N=173)	P value
Implantation rate (%)	40.6 (112/276)	47.1 (130/276)	0.123
Clinical pregnancy rate (%)	49.7 (86/173)	54.3 (94/173)	0.389
Clinical miscarriage rate (%)	4.6 (8/173)	6.4 (11/173)	0.479
Early pregnancy loss* rate (%)	8.7 (15/173)	11.6 (20/173)	0.373
Live birth rate (%)	40.0 (64/173)	45.1 (74/173)	0.351

*Biochemical pregnancies and clinical miscarriages combined

Table 3. Comparison of IVF-ET cycles outcomes between the studied groups

In the additional analysis of some of the other important parameters, no significant differences were noted between the groups.

Variable	Endometriosis group (N=173)	Tubal factor group (N=173)	P value
No. of oocytes retrieved (N)	11.2 ± 0.41	11.1 ± 0.39	0.773
No. of fertilized oocytes (N)	7.6 ± 0.31	7.5 ± 0.29	0.859
Fertilization rate (%)	69.4 ± 1.39	69.0 ± 1.38	0.847
Male factor present (%)	96 (55.5)	84 (48.6)	0.197

Table 4. Comparison of variables of IVF-ET cycles between the studied groups

2.3.2.2 Blastocyst quality and other possible predictors of various outcomes

The other objective of our investigation was to define the influence of blastocyst quality on various outcomes of IVF-ET cycles against all other important variables as controls in the group of women with endometriosis.

In our analysis, we incorporated 11 parameters as possible predictors of four main outcomes of stimulated IVF-ET cycles. The encompassed parameters were:

- patient's age,
- fertilization method (IVF or ICSI),
- type of gonadotrophin used for stimulation (human menopausal gonadotrophin (HMG) or recombinant follicle stimulation hormone (FSH)),
- number of retrieved oocytes,
- number of fertilized oocytes,
- fertilization rate,
- number of embryos on Day 2,
- number of blastocysts (embryos on Day 5),
- number of transferred blastocysts,
- number of frozen blastocysts and
- embryo quality score of transferred blastocysts.

Several examined predictors were transformed in categorical variables, as will be explained below. The six observed outcomes were:

- positive βhCG 14 days after ET,
- clinical pregnancy rate,
- live births rate,
- biochemical pregnancy rate,
- early clinical miscarriage rate, and
- early pregnancy loss rate (EPL - biochemical pregnancies and early clinical miscarriages taken together).

The relationship between continuous predictors and the number of implanted blastocysts was analyzed using Spearman correlation, while the effect of categorical predictors on the number of implanted blastocysts was tested by Mann-Whitney test or Kruskal-Wallis one-way analysis of variance. For all other outcome variables, the effect of possible predictors was analyzed using univariate logistic regression model. Before the incorporation of possible predictors in the multiple regression model, correlations among variables were tested to detect possible multicolinearity and to choose appropriate variables for the final analysis. The impact of possible predictors on the number of live born infants was evaluated using analysis of variance or chi-squared test, as appropriate. For post-hoc comparison of continuous variables, Bonferroni correction of alpha was used, while Keppel modification of Bonferroni correction was used for categorical variables.

Because of the low number of events per variables (EPV) for early clinical miscarriages, biochemical pregnancies and EPLs included in the logistic regression (Vittinghoff & McCulloch, 2007), a multiple model for analyzing the relative contribution of each predictor was constructed only for these three outcomes: **positive** βhCG 14 days following embryo transfer, clinical pregnancy rate and live births rate.

After testing all parameters for multicolinearity, a problem was detected in these pairs of variables: the number of retrieved oocytes/the number of fertilized oocytes, the number of retrieved oocytes/the number of embryos on Day 2, the number of fertilized oocytes/the number of embryos on Day 2 and the number of blastocysts/the number of frozen blastocysts. Accordingly, these pairs of variables were not included in the multiple regression model.

2.3.2.2.1 *Positive βhCG*

A univariate logistic regression model suggested a statistically significant correlation between the positive βhCG 14 days after ET and these indirect indicators of embryo quality: the number of embryos on Day 2 (OR=1.091; 95% CI 1.004 - 1.185, P<0.039), the number of blastocysts (OR=1.303; 95% CI 1.138 - 1.491, P<0.001), the number of frozen blastocysts (OR=1.436; 95% CI 1.208 - 1.708, P<0.001) and the embryo quality score of transferred blastocyst (in the form of two subgroups: the one with blastocysts of suboptimal quality only and the other with at least one blastocyst of optimal quality) (OR=5.339; 95% CI 2.782 - 10.246, P<0.001). A statistically significant correlation in univariate model was also noted for the age of the woman (OR=0.857; 95% CI 0.781 - 0.940, P=0.001), the number of retrieved oocytes (OR=1.069; 95% CI 1.006 - 1.135, P=0.030) and the number of fertilized oocytes (OR=1.088; 95% CI 1.003 - 1.180, P=0.041).

After controlling for the all other independent possible predictors in the multiple logistic regression model, the predictors of positive βhCG 14 days after ET in patients with endometriosis identified as statistically significant were the embryo quality score of transferred blastocyst (OR=4.278; 95% CI 1.976 - 9.265, P<0.001) and the age of the woman (OR=0.848; 95% CI 0.757 - 0.950, P=0.005).

2.3.2.2.2 *Clinical pregnancy rate*

Application of a logistic regression in univariate model showed that there was a statistically significant correlation between the clinical pregnancy rate and these indirect measures of embryo quality: the number of blastocysts (OR=1.278; 95% CI 1.122 - 1.457, P<0.001), the number of frozen blastocysts (OR=1.376; 95% CI 1.170 - 1.618, P<0.001) and the embryo quality score of transferred blastocyst (in the form of two subgroups: the one with blastocysts of suboptimal quality only and the other with at least one blastocyst of optimal quality) (OR=4.708; 95% CI 2.466 - 8.986, P<0.001). A statistically significant correlation in univariate model was also noted for the age of the woman (OR=0.875; 95% CI 0.781 - 0.941, P=0.001) and the number of retrieved oocytes (OR=1.069; 95% CI 1.007 - 1.134, P=0.027).

After controlling for all other independent possible predictors in the multiple logistic regression model, the predictors of the clinical pregnancy rate in patients with endometriosis identified as statistically significant were the embryo quality score (OR=3.485; 95% CI 1.608 - 7.553, P=0.002) and the age of the woman (OR=0.861; 95% CI 0.770 - 0.963, P=0.009).

2.3.2.2.3 *Live births*

A univariate logistic regression model indicated that there was a statistically significant correlation between the live births rate and these indirect measures of embryo quality: the number of blastocysts (OR=1.313; 95% CI 1.139 - 1.513, P<0.001), the number of frozen blastocysts (OR=1.402; 95% CI 1.183 - 1.661, P<0.001) and the embryo quality score of transferred blastocyst (in the form of two subgroups: the one with blastocysts of suboptimal quality only and the other with at least one blastocyst of optimal quality) (OR=3.316; 95% CI 1.693 - 6.496, P<0.001). A statistically significant correlation in univariate model was also noted for the age of the woman (OR=0.861; 95% CI 0.780 - 0.950, P=0.03).

After controlling for all other independent possible predictors in the multiple logistic regression model, the predictors of the live births rate in patients with endometriosis identified as statistically significant were the age of the woman (OR=0.851; 95% CI 0.756 - 0.958, P=0.07) and the number of frozen blastocysts (OR=1.319; 95% CI 1.034 - 1.683, P=0.026).

3. Conclusion

It is generally accepted that endometriosis and infertility are associated. However, the mechanisms connecting these complex conditions are still elusive. Results of different studies on virtually every aspect of this subject are controversial. Despite controversy, there is general agreement on relatively few final consequences of these pathophysiologic processes - endometriosis impairs the quality of oocytes with resulting lower fertilization rates and/or decreases implantation capacity of embryos (Pellicer et al., 2001).

One of indirect markers of oocyte quality and a possible predictor of embryo's implantation capacity is the quality of the developing embryo. As such, this parameter could be valuable for the assessment of influence of endometriosis on fertility of affected individuals. There are several indicators of embryo quality. Some of them are indirect measures of quality (the number of embryos on Day 2, the number of blastocysts, the number of frozen blastocysts, but also the implantation rate), while the only direct measure is the embryo quality score based on morphological characteristics of a developing embryo.

Our study showed no statistically significant difference of quality score of transferred blastocysts, indirect measures of embryo quality, common outcomes of IVF-ET cycles (implantation rate, clinical pregnancy rate, clinical miscarriage rate, early pregnancy loss rate and live births rate) or other analyzed parameters (male factor present, number of oocytes retrieved, number of fertilized oocytes, fertilization rate method of fertilization) between the group of infertile patients with endometriosis and the group with tubal factor infertility only.

In the further analysis of our data, we also showed that in infertile patients suffering only from endometriosis, embryo quality was a statistically significant positive predictor of positive βhCG measurement (if embryo quality was expressed in the form of embryo quality score, OR=4.278; 95% CI 1.976 - 9.265, P<0.001), clinical pregnancy rate (if embryo quality was expressed in the form of embryo quality score, OR=3.485; 95% CI 1.608 - 7.553, P=0.002) and live births rate (if embryo quality was expressed in the form of number of frozen blastocysts, OR=1.319; 95% CI 1.034 - 1.683, P=0.026). As expected, the patient's age was a statistically significant negative predictor of the success of IVF-ET cycles (positive βhCG measurement, clinical pregnancy rate and live births rate) in the observed group of patients.

Endometriosis is still an insufficiently explained condition. Numerous controversies still surrounding this complex disease indicate an obvious need for further clinical studies, meta-analyses and explanation of its pathophysiologic mechanisms. Should a consensus be reached on a precise methodology, future studies would definitely be more informative and results easier to use in clinical practice.

4. References

Arici, A.; Oral, E.; Bukulmez O.; Duleba, A.; Olive, DL. &, Jones, EE. (1996). The effect of endometriosis on implantation: results from the Yale University in vitro fertilization and embryo transfer program. *Fertil Steril*, 65: 603-7.

Barragán, JC.; Brotons, J.; Ruiz, JA. & Acien, P. (1992). Experimentally induced endometriosis in rats: effect on fertility and the effects of pregnancy and lactation on the ectopic endometrial tissue. *Fertil Steril*, 58: 1215–19.

Bergendal, A.; Naffah, S.; Nagy, C.; Bergqvist, A.; Sjöblom, P. & Hillensjö, T. (1998). Outcome of IVF in patients with endometriosis in comparison with tubal factor infertility. J Assist Reprod Genet, 15: 530-4.

Brizek, CL.; Schlaff, S.; Pellegrini, VA.; Frank, JB. & Worrilow, KC. (1995). Increased incidence of aberrant morphological phenotypes in human embryogenesis - an association with endometriosis. *J Assist Reprod Genet*, 12: 106-12.

Croxato, HB.; Ortiz, ME.; Guiloff, E.; Ibarra, A.; Salvatierra, AM.; Croxatto, HD. & Spilman, CH. (1978). Effect of 15 (S)-15-methyl prostaglandin F2a on human oviductal motility and ovum transport. *Fertil Steril*, 30: 408-14.

Damewood, MD.; Hesla, JS; Schlaff, WD.; Hubbard, M.; Gearhart, JD. & Rock, JA. (1990). Effect of serum from patients with minimal to mild endometriosis on mouse embryo development in vitro. *Fertil Steril*, 54: 917-20.

Dmowski, WP.; Radwanska, E.; Binor, Z. & Rana, N. (1986). Mild endometriosis and ovulatory dysfunction: effect of danazol treatment on success of ovulation induction. *Fertil Steril*, 46: 784-9.

Dmowski, WP.; Rana, N.; Michalowska, J.; Friberg, J.; Papierniak, C. & el-Roeiy. A. (1995). The effect of endometriosis, its stage and activity, and of auto antibodies on in vitro fertilization and embryo transfer success rates. *Fertil Steril*, 63: 555-62.

Dosen, M.; Vlaisavljevic, V. & Kovacic, B. (2011). Early miscarriage after single and double blastocyst transfer – An analysis of 1020 blastocyst transfers. Zdravniski Vestnik, 80: I-72-87.

Drake, TS. & Grunert, GM. (1980). The unsuspected pelvic factor in the infertility investigation. Fertil Steril, 34: 27–31.

Gardner, DK. & Schoolcraft, WB. (1999). In vitro culture of human blastocysts. In: Toward Reproductive Certainty: Fertility and Genetics Beyond, Jansen, R. & Mortimer, D., pp. 378-88, Partenon Publishing UK, Carnforth

Garrido, N.; Navarro, J.; Remohi, J.; Simon, C. & Pellicer, A. (2000). Follicular hormonal environment and embryo quality in women with endometriosis. Hum Reprod Update, 6; 67-74.

Grant, A. (1966). Additional sterility factors in endometriosis. Fertil Steril, 17: 514-9.

Hammond, MG.; Jordan, S. & Sloan, CS. (1986). Factors affecting pregnancy rates in donor insemination program using frozen semen. Am J Obstet Gynecol, 155: 480–5.

Harada, T.; Iwabe, T. & Terakawa, N. (2001). Role of cytokines in endometriosis. Fertil Steril, 76: 1-10.

Hasson, HM. (1976). Incidence of endometriosis in diagnostic laparoscopy. J Reprod Med, 16: 135–8.

Hourvitz, A.; Lerner-Geva, L.; Elizur, SE.; Baum, M.; Levron, J. & David B. (2006). Role of embryo quality in predicting early pregnancy loss following assisted reproductive technology. RBM Online, 13(4): 504–9.

Hunter, MI.; Huang, A. & DeCherney, AH. (2004). Endometriosis and ART. In: Textbook of Assisted Reproductive Techniques. Laboratory and Clinical Perspectives, Gardner, DK.; Weissman, A.; Howles, CM. & Shoham Z., pp. 761-9, Taylor & Francis UK, London.

Kovacic, B.; Vlaisavljevic, V.; Reljic, M. & Cizek-Sajko M. (2004). Developmental capacity of different morphological types of day human morulae and blastocysts. RBM Online, 8: 687–94.

Kovacic, B.; Cizek Sajko, M. & Vlaisavljevic, V. (2010). A prospective, randomized trial on the effect of atmospheric versus reduced oxygen concentration on the outcome of intracytoplasmic sperm injection cycles. Fertil Steril, 94(2): 511-9.

Lambers, MJ.; Mager, E.; Goutbeek, J.; McDonnell, J.; Homburg, R. & Schats R. (2007). Factors determining early pregnancy loss in singleton and multiple implantations. Hum Reprod, 22: 275–9.

La Sala, GB.; Nicoli, A.; Villani, MT.; Gallinelli, A.; Nucera, G. & Blickstein, I. (2005). Spontaneous embryonic loss rates in twin and singleton pregnancies after transfer of top- versus intermediate-quality embryos. Fertil Steril, 84: 1602–5.

Mahadevan, MM.; Trounson, AO. & Leeton, JF. (1983). The relationship of tubal blockage, infertility of unknown cause, suspected male infertility and endometriosis to success of in vitro fertilization and embryo transfer. Fertil Steril, 40: 755-62.

Mahmood, TA. & Templeton, AA. (1991). Folliculogenesis and ovulation in infertile women with mild endometriosis. Hum Reprod, 6: 227–231.

Matson, PL. & Yovich, JL. (1986). The treatment of infertility associated with endometriosis by in vitro fertilization. Fertil Steril, 46: 432-4.

Muse, K.; Wilson, EA. & Jawar, MJ. (1982). Prolactin hyperstimulation in response to thyrotropin-releasing hormone in patients with endometriosis. *Fertil Steril*, 38: 419-22.

Pellicer, A.; Oliveira, N.; Ruiz, A.; Remohí, J. & Simón, C. (1995). Exploring the mechanism(s) of endometriosis-related infertility: an analysis of embryo development and implantation in assisted reproduction. *Hum Reprod*, 10(Suppl 2): 91-7.

Pellicer, A.; Navarro, J.; Bosch, E.; Garrido, N.; Garcia-Velasco, JA.; Remohí, J. & Simón C. (2001). Endometrial quality in infertile women with endometriosis. *Ann N Y Acad Sci*, 943: 122-30.

Schenken, RS. &, Asch, RH. (1980). Surgical induction of endometriosis in the rabbit: effects on fertility and concentrations of peritoneal fluid prostaglandins. *Fertil Steril*, 34: 581-7.

Schenken, RS.; Asch, RH.; Williams, RF & Hodgen GD. (1984). Etiology of infertility in monkeys with endometriosis: luteinized unruptured follicle, luteal phase defects, pelvic adhesions and spontaneous abortions. *Fertil Steril*, 41: 122-30.

Steer, CV.; Mills, CL.; Tan, SL.; Campbell, S. & Edwards, RG. (1992). The cumulative embryo score: a predictive embryo scoring technique to select the optimal number of embryos to transfer in an in-vitro fertilization and embryo transfer programme. *Hum Reprod*, 7: 117-9.

Strathy, JH.; Molgaard, CA; Coulam, CB. & Melton, LJ. (1982). Endometriosis and infertility: A laparoscopic study of endometriosis among fertile and infertile women. *Fertil Steril*, 38: 667-72.

Soldati, G.; Piffaretti-Yanez, A.; Campana, A.; Marchini, M.; Luerti, M. & Balerna, M. (1989). Effect of peritoneal fluid on sperm motility and velocity distribution using objective measurements. *Fertil Steril*, 52: 113-9.

Tanbo, T.; Omland, A.; Dale, PO. & Abyholm, T. In vitro fertilization/embryo transfer in unexplained infertility and minimal peritoneal endometriosis. (1995). *Acta Obstet Gynecol Scand*, 74: 539-43.

The American Fertility Society. Revised American Fertility Society classification of endometriosis. (1985). *Fertil Steril*, 43: 351-2.

Tummon, IS.; Maclin, VM.; Radwanska, E.; Binor, Z. & Dmowski, WP. (1988). Occult ovulatory dysfunction in women with minimal endometriosis or unexplained infertility. *Fertil Steril*, 50: 716-20.

Vernon, MW. & Wilson, EA. (1985). Studies on the surgical induction of endometriosis in the rat. *Fertil Steril*, 44: 684-94.

Vittinghoff, E. & McCulloch, CE. (2007). Relaxing the rule of ten events per variable in logistic and Cox regression. *Am J Epidemiol*, 165(6): 710-8.

Winter, E.; Wang, J.; Davies, MJ. & Norman, R. (2002). Early pregnancy loss following assisted reproductive technology treatment. *Hum Reprod*, 17: 3220-3.

Yanushpolsky, EH.; Best, CL.; Jackson, KV.; Clarke, RN.; Barbieri, RL. & Hornstein, MD. (1998). Effects of endometriomas on oocyte quality, embryo quality and pregnancy rates in in vitro fertilization cycles: a prospective, case-controlled study. *J Assist Reprod Genet*, 15: 193-7.

Yeh, J. & Seibel, MM. (1987). Artificial insemination with donor sperm: A review of 108 patients. Obstet Gynecol, 70: 313–6.

Yovich, JL.; Yovich, JM.; Tuvik, AI.; Matson, PL. & Willcox DL. (1985). In-vitro fertilization for endometriosis. *Lancet*, 2(8454): 552.

Section 2

Diagnosis and Treatment

8

Current Insights and Future Advances in Endometriosis Diagnostics

Michele Cioffi and Maria Teresa Vietri
Department of General Pathology,
Faculty of Medicine and Surgery of Second University of Naples, Naples,
Italy

1. Introduction

Endometriosis is a benign gynaecological disease characterized by the presence of endometrial glands and stroma outside the uterine cavity. This condition is mainly found in women of reproductive age, from all ethnic and social groups and it is associated with pelvic pain and infertility. Endometriosis is typically present in the pelvis such as on the ovaries and pelvic peritoneum, but may also involve the bowel, ureter or bladder. It regresses after menopause or ovariectomy, suggesting it could depend on the production and metabolism of sex steroids: high concentrations of estrogens were found in the endometriotic lesions, which grow and regress in an oestrogen-dependent way. Nevertheless, the pathogenesis and the molecular mechanism that underlie the development of endometriosis have troubled the investigators through many years, remaining an enigma. The disease is widely accepted to result from the ectopic implantation of refluxed menstrual tissues. In addition, immunologic changes, environmental, hormonal and genetic factors contribute to the multifactorial etiology of endometriosis.

Many studies are therefore focusing on identifying markers for the diagnosis and follow-up of endometriosis. Although the "gold standard" for the diagnosis of endometriosis is the laparoscopy, many reports have suggested that various serum, peritoneal fluid and tissue markers might be associated with endometriosis. In fact, the identification of more sensitive and specific markers of endometriosis should facilitate the development of accurate and non-invasive techniques for diagnosis and prognosis (Table 1). Furthermore, the inheritable susceptibility to endometriosis justifies the growing interest in identifying genes and/or genetic polymorphisms that could lead to an increased risk of disease. Identifying these polymorphisms may open to their use as genetic biomarkers of endometriosis.

Over the last 20 years, several proteomics technologies have been used to research novel proteins with a potential etiological role in endometriosis, and to identify candidate serum markers for this condition. While some molecules identified by proteomics technologies may have a relevant role in the pathogenesis of endometriosis, the research of potential serum markers for this condition is still far from any clinical application.

The early diagnosis of endometriosis could prevent the possible progression of endometriosis, resulting in more pain, infertility and in a declining quality of life.

For a clinical purpose, the identification of highly sensitive and specific diagnostic test of endometriosis should facilitate the development of accurate and non-invasive test diagnosis and prognosis.

PERITONEAL FLUID AND/OR SERUM MARKERS	Glycoproteins
	Growth factors
	Cytokines
	Autoantibodies
	Hormones
	Proteolytic enzymes and their inhibitors
	Soluble adhesion molecules
	Environmental contaminant
ENDOMETRIAL MARKERS	Cell adhesion molecules (CAMs)
	Proteolytic enzymes
ENDOMETRIAL TISSUE BIOCHEMICAL MARKERS	Aromatase P450
	Hormone receptors
GENETIC MARKERS	Survivin gene expression
	p53 mutations
	Polymorphisms

Table 1. Markers for endometriosis

2. Peritoneal fluid and/or serum markers

Many serum and peritoneal fluid markers can be used to discriminate between patients with or without endometriosis (Table 2). Using markers with a high degree of sensitivity and specificity for endometriosis it is possible the development of peritoneal fluid and /or serum based diagnostics tools, therapeutic strategies and prognosis markers.

GLYCOPROTEINS	CA125
	CA19-9
GROWTH FACTORS	Hepatocyte growth factor (SF/HGF)
	Fibroblast growth factor (FGF)
	Epidermal growth factor (EGF)
	Transforming growth factor-alpha (TGF-α)
	Transforming growth factor-beta (TGF-β)
	Vascular endothelial growth factor (VEGF)
	Epidermal growth factor receptor (EGF-R)
	Insulin-like growth factor I (IGF-I)
CYTOKINES	TNF-α
	IL-1
	IL-6
	IL-8
	Monocyte chemoattractant protein (MCP)-1
	Interferon-γ

Table 2. Peritoneal fluid (PF) and/or serum markers for endometriosis

AUTOANTIBODIES	Antiendometrial antibodies
	Autoantibodies to oxidized lipoproteins
	Thyroid peroxidase antibodies
	IgG anti-laminin-1 antibodies
	Anti-phospholipid antibodies
HORMONES	Luteinizing hormone (LH)
	Progesterone
	Estradiol
	Thyroid stimulating hormone (TSH)
	Follicle stimulating hormone (FSH)
	Leptin
PROTEOLYTIC ENZYMES AND THEIR INHIBITORS	Matrix metalloproteinases (MMPs)
	Tissue inhibitors for MMPs (TIMPs)
SOLUBLE ADHESION MOLECULES	Intercellular adhesions molecule-1 (sICAM-1)
	Human leukocyte class I antigens (sHLA-I)
	E-cadherin
ENVIRONMENTAL CONTAMINAT	Dioxin-like chemicals

Table 2. Peritoneal fluid (PF) and/or serum markers for endometriosis. (Continuation)

2.1 Glycoproteins

Some serum glycoproteins, more commonly known for its use in the diagnosis or monitoring of cancers, might also serve as a marker for endometriosis, although levels are usually elevated only in advanced stages and are therefore not suitable for routine screening.

2.1.1 CA125

CA125 is a 200,000 Da glycoprotein expressed on the surface of the coelomic epithelium, including the epithelium of the endocervix, endometrium, fallopian tube, pelvic peritoneum and placental tissues. Serum CA125 levels increase in patients with malignant and benign gynaecologic diseases, including endometriosis.

Despite the most important clinical use of CA125 is the monitoring of patients with ovarian cancer, high levels can be found in women with endometriosis. Many studies have assessed the role of CA125 serum levels in women affected with endometriosis. The sensitivity and specificity of serum CA125 assay varies with the stage of disease. Usually, high CA125 serum levels can be found both in most patients with advanced endometriosis and in few patients with early-stage disease. Therefore, the routine use of serum CA125 cannot be used as a diagnostic tool for endometriosis. Serum CA125 may be more useful in evaluating recurrent disease or the outcome of a surgical treatment. CA125 levels may also be useful in patients with advanced endometriosis and several studies have suggested the use of this marker in the preoperative diagnosis of endometriosis.

The patients with endometriosis often undergo repeated laparoscopic examinations to assess the progress during and after therapy or to determine the recurrence of disease. Therefore, CA125 may be useful in the management of endometriosis and some authors suggest its assessment in women with suspected endometriosis, in association with laparoscopy and biopsy. In addition, in literature was reported that measurement of serum CA125 levels might be useful in identifying patients with infertility that may have severe endometriosis and could benefit from early surgical treatment.

CA125 levels were assessed in the PF of patients with and without endometriosis. Although levels of CA125 in the PF were almost 10 times higher than serum levels, no differences were found between women with and without endometriosis. In addition, CA125 levels are measured also in other body fluids, such as menstrual discharge and the uterine fluid, but are not useful in clinical practice.

2.1.2 CA19-9

CA19-9 is a high-molecular-weight glycoprotein that was initially thought to be an oncofetal antigen. Serum CA19-9 levels were elevated in patients with some malignant tumour, such as gastrointestinal adenocarcinoma, pancreatic carcinoma, or lung carcinoma; thus, the measurement of serum CA19-9 levels is useful in the diagnosis of these tumours. In gynaecology, the serum CA19-9 levels are elevated in patients with malignant and benign ovarian tumours. Furthermore, a case of an ovarian chocolate cyst with a markedly elevated serum CA19-9 level has been reported. In addition, it has been reported that serum CA19-9 levels in women with endometriosis are significantly reduced during therapy compared with the basal levels before treatment. Serum CA19-9 levels in patients with endometriosis are significantly higher than those in patients without endometriosis and that serum CA19-9 levels increase in accordance with the advancement of the clinical stage of endometriosis. CA19-9 was also detected in the endometrial glandular epithelium in ovarian chocolate cysts by immunohistochemistry. These results reveal that the measurement of the serum CA19-9 levels, as well as the serum CA125 level, may prove to be a valuable tool for predicting the severity of endometriosis as diagnosed by laparoscopy.

2.2 Growth factors

The endometrium in endometriosis behaves like tumorous tissue and the growth factors involved in tumour proliferation, angiogenesis and invasiveness have been investigated for their expression in endometriosis. Indeed, the degree of endometriosis is positively correlated with the concentration in peritoneal fluid and serum of *Hepatocyte Growth Factor/Scatter Factor (HGF/SF)*, a multifunctional polypeptide that has been implicated in embryo development, tissue repair, and cancer growth, produced mainly by mesenchymal cells with activity mediated through the c-met receptor found principally on epithelial and endothelial cells (Zong et al., 2003).

Inflammatory macrophages and the inflammatory mediators they release could be related to the ectopic implantation of endometriosis: *Fibroblast Growth Factor (FGF)*, *Epidermal Growth Factor (EGF)*, *Transforming Growth Factor-alpha (TGF-α)*, *Transforming Growth Factor-beta (TGF-β) and Tumor Necrosis Factor-alpha (TNF- α)*. It is been shown that these growth factors stimulate in vitro proliferation of endometrial stromal cells, suggesting that they could improve the implantation of endometrial cells.

Elevated serum levels of *Epidermal Growth Factor Receptor (EGF-R)*, involved in angiogenesis, suggest an active role for EGF in the development of endometriosis (Matalliotakis et al., 2003a, 2003b).

Insulin-like Growth Factor I (IGF-I) serum levels in patients with early stage endometriosis, and in healthy control, were significantly lower than the levels in patients with late stage endometriosis, suggesting that IGF-I is an important mediator in the development and/or maintenance of endometriosis or progression to late stage disease (Gurgan et al., 1999).

Many studies report that angiogenesis is probably involved in the pathogenesis of endometriosis. *Vascular endothelial growth factor (VEGF)*, also known as vascular permeability factor, is one of the most potent and specific angiogenic factors. VEGF has emerged as an important regulator of normal angiogenesis and pathological neovascularisation.

VEGF levels in both peritoneal fluid and serum were higher in women with endometriosis compared with controls. The cellular source of VEGF in peritoneal fluid has not yet been precisely defined. Some evidence suggests that the endometriotic lesions themselves produce this factor and that the activated peritoneal macrophages are able to synthesize and secrete VEGF (Matalliotakis et al., 2003a, 2003b).

2.3 Immunological markers

The immune system plays an important role in the pathogenesis of endometriosis, which begins, therefore, to be treated as an autoimmune disease. T-helper, T-suppressor and natural killer (NK) cells concentrations are altered in serum and peritoneal fluid of patients with endometriosis (Lebovic et al., 2001; Nothnick, 2001). In addition, IgG and IgA anti-endometrial antibodies have been detected in the sera and vaginal and cervical secretions of endometriosis patients. The presence of anti-phospholipids and anti-histones antibodies has been documented by some authors and questioned by others. These observations would believe that markers of immune reactivity, particularly cytokines, might be used as a diagnostic aid for endometriosis.

2.3.1 Cytokines

Macrophages are a major source of many cytokines involved in immune response, haematopoiesis, inflammation and many other homeostatic processes. Upon stimulation by microorganisms, microbial products or endogenous factors including cytokines, macrophages can *de novo* synthesize and release a large variety of cytokines (i.e. IL-1, IL-1ra, IL-6, IL-8, IL-10, IL-12, TNF-α, IFN-α, IFN-γ, MCP-1, MCP-3, MIF, M-CSF, G-CSF, GM-CSF, MIP-1, MIP-2, LIF, OSM, TGF-β). Some cytokines can up-regulate the production of cytokines by macrophages (IL-3, GM-CSF, IFN-γ) while others can inhibit it (IL-4, IL-10, IL-13, TGF-β). In addition, these cytokines can modulate most of the macrophage functions and cell surface marker expression. Other cytokines (chemokines such as MCP-1, 2, 3, MIP-1,2 and RANTES) contribute to the recruitment of circulating monocytes within tissues.

T lymphocytes are important regulatory cells that secrete several cytokines and participate actively in this inflammatory response. According to the pattern of cytokines secreted, the immune response is classified as cytotoxic or type 1 (IFN-γ, IL-2, IL-12) and humoral or type 2 (IL-4, IL-5, IL-10 and IL-13) (Barcelò et al., 2006).

The role of cytokines and growth factors in the pathophysiology of endometriosis is evident. They are probably responsible for the proliferation of endometrial cells and implantation of endometrial cells or tissue. In addition, cytokines increase the tissue remodelling through their influence on matrix metalloproteinases. Probably the most important effect of cytokines on ectopic endometrial tissue is an increase in angiogenesis of ectopic endometrial tissue and neovascularisation of the affected region. Therefore, cytokines play an important role in the initiation, propagation and regulation of immune and inflammation responses. The activation of immune cells results in a burst and cascade of inflammatory cytokines.

ELISA kits are available to assess the cytokines in the serum and peritoneal fluid (PF) of endometriosis patients. PF is rich with variable cellular components including macrophages, mesothelial cells, lymphocytes, eosinophils and mastcells. Approximately 85% of PF leukocytes are macrophages. It has been hypothesized that peritoneal macrophage activation is a key step in disease initiation and progression. Activated macrophages in the peritoneal cavity of women with endometriosis are potent producers of cytokines (Bedaiwy et al., 2002). Thus, PF contains a rich mixture of cytokines. Cytokines, such as TNF-α, IL-1, IL-6, IL-8, monocyte chemoattractant protein (MCP)-1 and IFN-γ, are elevated in the PF of women with endometriosis, suggesting that they are involved in the progression of the disease. The level of IL-1 in PF is positively correlated with the progression of endometriosis, but the serum level of IL-1 seems to have no correlation with endometriosis.

The Tumor Necrosis Factors (TNF) superfamily of cytokines represents a multifunctional group proinflammatory cytokines, which activate signalling pathways for cell survival, apoptosis, inflammatory responses, and cellular differentiation. Induction of cellular responses to TNF occurs through two receptors, TNFR1 (TNF Receptor-1 or CD120a) and TNFR2 (TNF Receptor-2 or CD120b). TNFR1 is activated in most human tissues by the binding of TNFα. On the other hand, TNFR2 is primarily expressed in immune cells and is activated by both TNFα and TNFβ (Kawasaki et al., 2002).

The main TNF is TNF-α, which is produced by neutrophils, activated lymphocytes, macrophages, NK cells and several non-hematopoietic cells. The TNF-α is involved in the normal physiology of the endometrial proliferation in the human endometrium. TNF-α is expressed predominantly in epithelial cells, especially in the secretory phase. The stromal cells stain for TNF-α mostly in the proliferative phase of the menstrual cycle. These data suggest that hormones influence the role of this cytokine.

Some reports found that concentrations of TNF-α in both serum and PF were very high at the early stage of the disease and decreased with the severity of the endometriosis. Moreover, the assessment of TNF-α levels in the PF can be used as a basis for non-surgical diagnosis of endometriosis.

The role of IL-6 in the pathogenesis of endometriosis has been widely studied. IL-6 is a regulator of inflammation and immunity, which may represent a physiological link between the endocrine and immune systems. IL-6 also modulates the secretion of other cytokines, promotes T-cell activation, differentiation of B cells and inhibits the growth of several human cell lines (Nothnick, 2001).

The data about IL-6 levels in the PF of patients with endometriosis are controversial. In fact, no statistically significant differences are reported between controls and endometriosis patients. In contrast, serum levels of IL-6 were significantly higher in women with endometriosis than in controls and the highest levels were found in women with chocolate cysts (Wieser et al., 2003; Iwabe et al., 2003).

2.3.2 Autoantibodies

Endometriosis is supposed to be an autoimmune disorder and many autoantibodies have been proposed as a diagnostic test. A variety of autoantibodies have been detected in endometriosis patients (thyroid peroxidase antibody, IgG anti-laminin-1 antibodies, anti-phospholipid antibodies and the novel anti-PDIK1L antibodies). The most commonly reported types are antiendometrial antibodies, autoantibodies against the oxidative-stress-induced, antigens to malondialdehyde-modified low-density lipoprotein (LDL) and oxidized low-density lipoprotein (Ox-LDL).

Some investigators have hypothesized that antiendometrial antibodies may cause infertility in some women with endometriosis by preventing the fertilized embryo from implanting in the uterus. In addition, increasing evidence suggests that oxidative stress occurs in the PF of women with endometriosis and oxidatively modified lipoproteins were found in the PF.

2.4 Hormones

Serum and PF hormones levels vary in patients affected with endometriosis. Luteinizing hormone (LH) levels are significantly higher in both serum and PF in patients with endometriosis than in normal controls (Illera et al., 2001). However, levels of prolactin, thyroid stimulating hormone (TSH) and follicle stimulating hormone (FSH) in the serum were no different between the different groups.

Recently it was reported that serum concentrations of leptin are increased in patients with endometriosis. This increase may play an anti-apoptotic role in activated endometrial stromal cells into the peritoneal cavity, stimulating endometrial cell implantation and cause infertility (Tanaka et al., 2003). Furthermore another study measured the serum concentration of leptin using a radioimmunoassay method, showing a significant association between leptin concentrations and stage of endometriosis (Viganò et al., 2002).

2.5 Proteolytic enzymes and their inhibitors

The physiological changes in endometriosis involve multiple steps of matrix remodelling. Endometriosis associated to abnormal matrix remodelling is affected by several molecular factors including proteolytic enzymes and their inhibitors, which mediate tissue turnover, and ovarian steroids, which normally regulate reconstruction of endometrium in the menstrual cycle.

The extracellular matrix (ECM) constitutes a well-organized network structure that surrounds the cells. The tissue remodelling involving ECM turnover is regulated by the pooled action of proteolytic enzymes, matrix metalloproteinases (MMP) and tissue inhibitors for MMP (TIMP). The inappropriate expression of MMP and TIMP is associated with tumorigenesis and metastasis, as well as with endometriosis.

Several MMP have been implicated in the development of endometriosis (Sillem et al., 2001). The levels of MMP and TIMP in patients with endometriosis are different depending on the method of measurement and collection of samples of different tissues at different stages of endometriosis. The values of TIMP-1 is determined by radioimmunoassay measurement in serum of patients with PF in endometriosis are lower than in controls. In contrast, the concentration of TIMP-1 was restored after treatment with gonadotropin releasing hormone. Another study reported that there was no significant difference in levels of cathepsin D, a proteolytic enzyme thought to promote digestion of ECM proteins in endometriosis, in serum from women with and without endometriosis.

2.6 Soluble adhesion molecules

It is thought that the retrograde flow of the menstrual debris to the peritoneal cavity plays an important role in the origin of endometriosis but the mechanism of endometrial cells implantation remains unknown. Recently many studies have reported the importance of adhesion molecules in this process.

Several adhesion molecules (CAM) are expressed in the human endometrium: i.e. integrins, cadherins and immunoglobulin superfamilies. These adhesion molecules show cyclical changes during the menstrual cycle. The major cell surface receptors of the ECM are the *integrins* that contain large (α) and small (β) subunits.

β1-integrins are known to mediate the interaction between the cell-cell and cell-extracellular matrices and are represented by very late activation (VLA) antigen molecules. It is well known that endometriosis is frequently associated with immunological abnormalities. However, only a few studies have been conducted on the adhesion molecules, particularly on β 1-integrins, in endometriosis. It has reported that integrins are expressed in the endometrium in endometriosis. The ability of endometriotic tissues to express integrins may explain the high recurrence rates in patients with endometriosis, as these samples retain their adhesion potency after retrograde menstruation and are thus able to establish cell-cell and cell-matrix interactions with the surrounding peritoneum.

The soluble forms of the *intercellular-adhesion molecule-1 (sICAM-1)* are secreted from the endometrium and endometriotic implants. Moreover, endometrium from women with endometriosis secretes a higher amount of this molecule than tissue from women without the disease. Consequently, a strong correlation exists between levels of sICAM-1 and the number of endometriotic implants in the pelvis. Therefore, it has been hypothesized that sICAM-1 may be useful in the diagnosis of endometriosis (Leng et al., 2002). Many investigators have reported a significant increase in serum concentration of sICAM-1 in patients with endometriosis. The sICAM-1 concentrations were higher in patients with stage I–II endometriosis, suggesting that studies on these soluble adhesion molecules can help clarify the pathogenic mechanisms of endometriosis. Elevated ICAM-1 levels were found in patients with severe endometriosis, but its sensitivity is not high and the concomitant use of the CA125 marker increases the sensitivity and specificity of detection (Somigliana et al., 2002).

The **E-cadherin** mediates cell-cell interaction and cells adhere preferentially to cells that express the same cadherin. Cadherins are distributed widely among animals and play a potentially significant role in morphogenetic events during embryogenesis. Cadherin is also expressed in the cell-to-cell boundaries of the endometrium. It is reported that E-cadherin expression on the endometrium was higher in the secretory phase than in the proliferative phase, although there is one report that the expression was unchanged during the cycle. Furthermore, the level of E-cadherin in serum of endometriosis patients was significantly higher than that of control group.

The level of E-cadherin in the serum of both III stage and IV stage endometriosis patients was higher than that of I and II stage patients. However, the difference between them was not statistically significant. E-cadherin may play a role on the morbidity of endometriosis and the serum E-cadherin assay might be helpful as a serum marker for the diagnosis and management of endometriosis (Fu & Lang, 2002).

2.7 Environmental contaminant

Environmental toxins, such as dioxins and polychlorinated biphenyls are some of the factors that have been suggested to play a significant role in the development of endometriosis. In fact, detection of environmental contaminant residues in serum and ovarian follicular fluid confirms this hypothesis. Dioxin-like chemicals, such as 2,3,7,8-tetrachlorodibenzo-p-dioxin (TCDD) and polyhalogenated aromatic hydrocarbons (PHAHs), may exert effects on the pathophysiology of endometriosis through a number of pathways: (1) activation of pro-carcinogens; (2) altered synthesis and metabolism of estradiol; (3) altered production of pro-inflammatory growth factors or cytokines and (4) alterations in tissue remodelling processes.

Exposure to HAHs and TCDD seems to be associated with a dose-dependent increase in the incidence and severity of endometriosis. TCDD may target peripheral blood and peritoneal and endometrial leukocyte populations inducing chronic expression of TNF-α and other inflammatory mediators resulting in increased adhesion, vascularization and proliferation of endometriotic cells. It has been suggested that an elevated concentration of TNF-a might participate in TCDD-mediated toxicity and contribute to the pathogenesis of endometriosis.

Dioxins may affect the expression of TNF-α via the induction of an inflammatory cytokine network, since the region of DNA that recognize the ligand-activated AhR, the dioxin-response element of DRE, is present in the genes of potent inducers of TNF-α including IL-1b, IL-6 and IFN-γ (Rier & Foster, 2003).

3. Endometrial markers

The adhesion of endometrial cells to the extracellular matrix (ECM) would be expected to play a central role in the pathogenesis of endometriosis. Various cell adhesion molecules (CAMs) have been investigated for their expression in endometriotic endometrium. Each cell type expresses a distinct pattern of integrins and other CAMs, including the cadherins, selectins and members of the immunoglobulin family that determines cell shape, maintains cell position and polarity and affects hormonal responsiveness. In addition, apoptosis might be mediated through loss of appropriate signals from the ECM through alternations in the integrin expression. Based on cell adhesion and the genes involving in adhesion and invasion aspects, cell adhesion molecules (CaMs) and proteolytic enzymes were investigated for their mechanisms in association with the progression of endometriosis.

4. Endometrial tissue biochemical markers

4.1 Aromatase P450

Aromatase P450 is the key enzyme for biosynthesis of oestrogen, which is an essential hormone for the establishment and growth of endometriosis. There is no detectable aromatase enzyme activity in normal endometrium; therefore, oestrogen is not locally produced in endometrium. Endometriosis tissue, however, contains very high levels of aromatase enzyme, which leads to production of significant quantities of oestrogen (Dheenadayalu et al., 2002). Moreover, one of the best-known mediators of inflammation and pain, prostaglandin E2 (PGE2), was found to be the most potent known inducer of aromatase activity in endometriotic stromal cells. The clinical significance of local aromatase activity that is induced strikingly by PGE2 in endometriotic tissue was exemplified recently by the successful use of an aromatase inhibitor to treat an unusually aggressive case of recurrent postmenopausal endometriosis that was resistant to any other surgical or hormonal modalities of treatment. Therefore, the aberrant expression of aromatase P450 in endometriotic tissue, in contrast to eutopic endometrium, justifies the local biosynthesis of estrogen that promotes the growth of these lesions and possibly mediates the resistance to conventional hormonal treatments, which is observed in a number of women with endometriosis. The molecular mechanisms that are responsible for aberrant aromatase P450 expression may provide insights into the etiology of endometriosis and lead to identification of molecular targets for the development of novel treatment strategies. Although endometrial aromatase P450 expression does not correlate with the disease stage, a recent study demonstrated that detection of aromatase P450 transcripts in the endometrium of endometriosis patients might be a potential qualitative marker of endometriosis.

4.2 Hormone receptors

The expression of receptors for the ovarian steroid hormones oestrogen and progesterone was studied immunohisto-chemically using monoclonal antibodies. The quantification of these receptors in the endometrium could be potentially useful in screening for this disease.

The eutopic endometrium of patients with endometriosis is different from endometrium of fertile controls regarding apoptosis, cytokines and other characteristics. Although cyclic changes were also detected in ectopic endometrium, different patterns of receptor expression suggested a difference in hormonal regulation between the two sites.

The concentrations of steroid receptors in ectopic endometrium increased gradually as the cycle progressed. Compared with eutopic endometrium, oestrogen and progesterone receptor concentrations were significantly lower in the proliferative phase, similar in the early secretory phase and significantly higher in the late secretory phase. The different patterns of receptor expression suggested different hormonal regulations between eutopic and ectopic endometrium.

There are two isoforms for oestrogen (ER) and progesterone (PR) receptors-ER-α and ER-β, PRA and PR-B. These isoforms exist in the endometrium and their function and content are different from one another. The different concentrations and biological activity of steroid receptor isoforms might lead to various hormonal responsiveness of ectopic endometrium. High concentrations of ER and PR in the ectopic endometrium during the secretory phase could explain the high proliferative activity of endometriotic tissue in this phase. Conversely, a decrease in ER and PR expression in ectopic implants during the secretory phase might lead to diminished proliferation. The expression of oestrogen and progesterone receptors may be regarded as an index of differentiation of the endometriotic implant. Consequently, ER and PR receptors may be used as markers of the activity of all subtypes of endometriotic lesions.

5. Genetic markers

Several genetic abnormalities or mutations have been suggested that might be related to endometriosis. Many technological approaches can help identify possible genetic markers of endometriosis. A number of technologies have emerged to facilitate progress in this direction (Taylor et al., 2002). Gene based technologies includes subtractive cDNA hybridization and cDNA microarray techniques.

5.1 Survivin gene expression

In endometriotic lesions, although derived from normal endometrium, decreased expression of adhesion molecules and increased expression of proteolytic enzymes may contribute to establishment of endometrial glands and stroma at ectopic sites, likely as behaviour of cancer cells. Normal epithelial cells undergo apoptosis when they separate from their primary tissue. However, spontaneous apoptosis of ectopic endometrial tissue is impaired in women with endometriosis, and its decreased susceptibility to apoptosis might participate in the growth, survival, and invasion of endometriotic tissue. Although there have been some reports on the induction of apoptosis in endometriotic lesions, there is no consensus on the mechanism of escape from apoptosis in endometriosis, and little is known on the correlation between survival activity and invasive phenotype in endometriotic cells. Among the regulators of cell death, inhibitor of apoptosis (IAP) proteins has recently emerged as modulators of an evolutionarily conserved step in apoptosis, which may potentially involve the direct inhibition of terminal effector caspases 3 and 7.

Survivin is a novel inhibitor of apoptosis and is expressed during fetal development and in cancer tissues, but its expression has not been reported in normal adult tissues or benign diseases. Survivin gene and protein expression was detected in normal human endometrium and that survivin could play an important role in physiological homeostasis during the normal menstrual cycle (Konno et al., 2000). The survivin is also expressed in ectopic endometriotic tissue; however, there has been no report on the biological significance of survivin in endometriosis, an aggressive tumour-like benign disease.

5.2 p53 mutations

Genomic alterations may represent important events in the development of endometriosis. Tumour suppressor genes play a role in the regulation of cell growth and prevention of carcinogenesis. The altered tumour suppressor genes might be related with the development of endometriosis. p53, a representative tumour suppressor, is involved in cell proliferation and progression of various tumour types (Akahane et al., 2007).

High frequency of p53 locus deletion was observed in the endometriosis specimens (Bischoff et al., 2002). The p53 protein abnormalities and chromosomal aberrations may be involved in malignant transformation of ovarian endometriosis (Mhawech et al., 2002). In contrast, some investigators have demonstrated the undetectable expression of p53 in the endometriosis specimens.

Although the real role of p53 polymorphism has not been clarified, it deserves more attentions in the study of endometriosis and the development of gene therapy. However, the real roles of these p53 gene polymorphisms upon endometriosis remain to be clarified. Lager cohort recruitment is request for its further clarification. After the elucidation of these issues, some tumour suppressor gene polymorphisms might become useful markers to predict the future development of endometriosis as well as the development and intervention of genetic therapy.

5.3 Polymorphisms

Some genetic polymorphisms, involved in sex steroids biosynthesis and metabolism, may be reasonably associated with an increased risk of endometriosis. Specific genes with polymorphisms have been investigated for an association with endometriosis. Some association studies implicated GALT (a gene involved in galactose metabolism) and GSTM1 and NAT2 (genes encoding for the detoxification enzymes) as possible disease susceptibility genes. Recent finding have added to the evidence for the involvement of GSTM1 and NAT2, but have cast doubt on the role of GALT. The CDKN1A gene codon 31-arginine/serine polymorphism is not associated with endometriosis. Polymorphisms of the arylhydrocarbon receptor (AHR) gene and related genes were examined, and in at least one study, no association was found.

The endometriosis regresses after menopause or ovariectomy, suggesting it could depend on the production and metabolism of sex steroids (Kitawaki et al., 2002): high concentrations of estrogens were found in the endometriotic lesions, which grow and regress in an oestrogen-dependent way.

The inheritable susceptibility to endometriosis justifies the growing interest in identifying genes and/or genetic polymorphisms that could lead to an increased risk of disease. Identifying these polymorphisms may open to their use as genetic biomarkers of endometriosis (Vietri et al., 2007a, 2007b). Some genetic polymorphisms, involved in sex steroids biosynthesis and metabolism, may be reasonably associated with an increased risk of endometriosis, like progesterone receptor (PR), AR, oestrogen receptor (AR), 17beta-hydroxysteroid dehydrogenase type 1 (HSD17B1), cytochrome P450 subfamily 17 (CYP17) and cytochrome P450 subfamily 19 (CYP19) (Guo, 2006). No doubt this list is likely to increase over the years. The most widely used approach for the identification of endometriosis-predisposing genetic polymorphisms are the genetic association studies, by which genetic susceptibility polymorphisms are identified through the identification and assessment of the difference in allele/genotype frequencies between patients and control subjects.

The **CYP17 genotype** contains a single nucleotide T>C polymorphism situated 34bp upstream of the translation initiation site. C allele may have great promoter activity, increasing the transcription of P450c17 alpha enzyme. This effect amplifies the production of precursor androgens that are subsequently converted to estrogens. In fact, C allele is associated with high levels of estradiol in young women. CYP19 gene lies on chromosome 15 and encodes cytochrome P450, a major component of aromatase. Aromatase is a key enzyme in the conversion of androgens to estrogens, and mediates the rate-limiting step in the metabolism of C_{19} androgens to estrogens. Different polymorphisms of CYP19 are present in the gene and have been related to variations of aromatase activity (Gennari et al., 2004). A silent SNP, C1558T, corresponding to the 3' untraslated region of the mRNA, has been correlated to the level of aromatase mRNA in breast tumour cells. Another polymorphism, GA at Val80, has been previously associated with breast cancer risk. Few studies have been published on the association between CYP17 T>C polymorphism with risk of endometriosis, showing controversial data. Some studies connected C1558T polymorphism with endometriosis risk (Huber et al., 2005), while no report relates Val80 SNP to endometriosis.

The **CYP19 genotype** may play a role in increased risk of endometriosis lying on an environmental and genetic background. The polymorphisms of CYP19 are significantly represented in Val80 and C1558T in patients affected with endometriosis. Despite endometriosis is a multifactorial disease, identifying Val80 and C1558T polymorphisms of CYP19 could help to comprehend the mechanisms of endometriosis. The assessment of these polymorphisms could help to anticipate the diagnosis or expect it in asymptomatic women to elaborate a follow up program. Other than that, a follow up by ultrasound and blood markers could be proposed in these patients, in order to define unclear symptoms such as dysmenorrhoea and chronic pelvic pain.

6. Future scope

Endometriosis is associated with genetic and immunological influences and exposure to environmental factors. It seems to result from a complex sequence of events in which multiple gene loci interact with each other and the environment to produce the disease phenotype, but thus far little is known about the candidate genes involved (Balow & Kennedy 2005). Because of this complexity, endometriosis is ideally suited as a target for genome wide scanning. Mutations and single-nucleotide polymorphisms (SNPs) have been identified in a number of genes that might confer susceptibility to endometriosis, but their precise role remains to be determined.

Proteome analysis is now widely accepted as a complementary technology to genetic profiling and together enables a better understanding of diseases and the development of new treatments. Proteomics allows the simultaneous observation of alterations in protein expression that may be either a precursor to or causative in disease development or a consequence of the disease. These techniques check and identify proteins that are expressed differently in patients with endometriosis versus normal controls. More recently, protein arrays using antibodies enable the screening of thousands of proteins against one sample. In future, such arrays could measure the expressions of multiple proteins to reveal changes in their regulation and expression in disease states. Furthermore, by using protein chip arrays, differential analysis of protein expression in women with and without differential protein profiling technology can be developed into a powerful tool for endometriosis research.

The study of protein function and protein-protein interaction can clarify the biology of the disease more so than the application of genomics. This is because gene expression and biological effects are linked via complex protein synthesis and gene interaction pathways.

Genomics includes hybridization techniques (e.g. differential colony hybridization), subtractive techniques (e.g. hybridization and representational difference analysis), gel-based techniques (e.g. RNA arbitrarily primed or differential display), and sequencing based techniques (e.g. expression sequence tags and serial analysis of gene expression). Furthermore, the use of DNA microarrays allows the search for new gene expression markers of endometriosis by identifying differentially expressed genes in endometriosis implants compared with endometrial tissue. The aim of the technique is to identify changes in gene expression characterizing the disease state so that we can understand the disease's progression and identify novel therapeutic targets.

Apart from the better understanding of the pathophysiology and the metabolic pathways that lead to potential biomarkers for endometriosis, there are still issues to be clarified and applications to be achieved. Once a protein or small number of proteins have been shown to be differentially expressed in endometriosis, the next step will be to use this information to try to develop a non-invasive diagnostic test for endometriosis. This diagnostic test should ideally have good sensitivity and specificity as well as satisfactory positive and negative predicative values for the detection of endometriosis, and also be cost effective and readily available.

Genetic markers that are prognostic for endometriosis can be genotyped early in life and could predict individual response to various risk factors and treatment. Genetic predisposition revealed by genetic analysis for susceptibility genes can provide an integrated assessment of the interaction between genotypes and environmental factors, resulting in synergistically increased prognostic value of diagnostic tests. Thus, pre-symptomatic and early symptomatic genetic testing is expected to be the cornerstone of the paradigmatic shift from late surgical interventions to earlier preventative therapies. Thus, there is an urgent need for novel genetic markers that are predictive of endometriosis and endometriosis progression, particularly in treatment decisions for individuals who are recognized as having endometriosis.

Such genetic markers may enable prognosis of endometriosis in much larger populations compared with the populations that can currently be evaluated by using existing risk factors and biomarkers.

The availability of a genetic test may allow, for example, early diagnosis and prognosis of endometriosis, as well as clinical intervention to mitigate progression of the disease. The use of these genetic markers will also allow selection of subjects for clinical trials involving novel treatment methods.

The discovery of genetic markers associated with endometriosis will further provide novel targets for therapeutic intervention or preventive treatments of endometriosis and enable the development of new therapeutic agents for treating endometriosis.

7. Conclusions

One of the main objectives of the gynaecologist is to diagnose endometriosis without the use of laparoscopy or laparotomy. Currently, laparoscopy offers the most specific and sensitive technique for evaluating and monitoring endometriosis. Even so, microscopic or occult endometriosis may be misdiagnosed because of the inability to visualize some lesions. Attempts for early diagnosis and treatments of endometriosis have been weighed down by lack of proper methods to study and manage the disease. Furthermore, the need for non-invasive diagnostic methods is evident because the laparoscopy is a surgical procedure with potentially dangerous risks.

At present, there are no reliable markers for the diagnosis and prognosis of endometriosis and identification of serum and endometrial markers is decisive for disease diagnosis and follow-up of patients.

The diagnostic laboratories are using new genomic and proteomic technologies to develop novel diagnostic and therapeutic approaches for endometriosis. These technologies will facilitate the generation of molecular expression profiles and then identifying potential gene and protein targets. This will lead to available markers with high sensitivity and specificity for screening of endometriosis, then to the development of serum diagnostic tools, therapeutic strategies and prognosis markers.

The combination of immunological discoveries and recent advances in DNA technologies may provide the long sought screening tool with the desirable diagnostic accuracy for this puzzling disorder.

The identification of specific genetic alterations and protein profiles associated with endometriosis offers a unique opportunity to develop assays for early diagnosis and/or treatment. By identifying proteins in biological samples, a minimally invasive tool should be feasible to assess the presence of disease and monitor response to treatment and/or disease progression.

The promise for gene-based diagnostic tests for endometriosis and rational development of genetically targeted and molecular therapeutic strategies is, in principle, excellent. The evolving genomic and proteomic technologies remain poised to revolutionize the diagnosis and treatment of endometriosis, but have not yet lead to a single new therapy or tested biomarker. Many problems remain to be resolved and, while some of these are technical in nature, the most intractable ones have mainly to do with the complex and multifactorial character of the disease itself.

8. References

Akahane, T., Sekizawa, A., Purwosunu, Y., Nagatsuka, M. & Okai, T. (2007). The role of p53 mutation in the carcinomas arising from endometriosis, *Int J Gynecol Pathol*, Vol. 26, No. 3, (July 2007), pp. 345-351, ISSN 0277-1691

Balow, D.H. & Kennedy, S. (2005). Endometriosis: new genetic approaches and therapy, *Ann Rev Med*, Vol. 56, pp. 345-356, ISSN 0066-4219

Barcelò, B., Pons, J., Fuster, A., Sauleda, J., Noguera, A., Ferrer, J.M. & Agustì, A.G. (2006). Intracellular cytokine profile of T lymphocytes in patients with chronic obstructive pulmonary disease, *Clin Exp Immunol*, Vol. 145, No. 3, (September 2006), pp. 474-479, ISSN 0009-9104

Bedaiwy, M.A., Falcone, T., Sharma, R.K., Goldberg, J.M., Attaran, M., Nelson, D.R. & Agarwal A. (2002). Prediction of endometriosis with serum and peritoneal fluid markers: a prospective controlled trial, *Hum Reprod,* Vol. 17, No. 2, (March 2002), pp. 426-431, ISSN 0268-1161

Bischoff, F.Z., Heard, M. & Simpson, J.L. (2002). Somatic DNA alterations in endometriosis: high frequency of chromosome 17 and p53 loss in late-stage endometriosis, *J Reprod Immunol,* Vol. 55, No. 1-2, (May-June 2002), pp. 49-64, ISSN 0165-0378

Dheenadayalu, K., Mak, I. Gordts, S., Campo, R., Higham, J., Puttemans, P.; White, J., Christian, M., Fusi, L. & Brosens J. (2002). Aromatase P450 messenger RNA expression in eutopic endometrium is not a specific marker for pelvic endometriosis, *Fertil Steril,* Vol. 78, No. 4 (October 2002), pp. 825–829, ISSN 0015-0282

Fu, C. & Lang, J. (2002). Serum soluble E-cadherin level in patients with endometriosis, *Chin Med Sci J,* Vol. 17, No. 2, (June 2002), pp. 121–123, ISSN 1001-9294

Gennari, L., Nuti, R., & Bilezikian, J.P. (2004). Aromatase activity and bone homeostasis in men, *J Clin Endocrinol Metab,* Vol. 89, No. 12, (December 2004), pp. 5898-5907, ISSN 0021-972X

Guo, S.W. (2006). Association of endometriosis risk and genetic polymorphisms involving sex steroid biosynthesis and their receptors: a meta-analysis, *Gynecol Obstet Invest,* Vol. 61, No. 2, pp. 90-105, ISSN 0378-7346

Gurgan, T., Bukulmez, O., Yarali, H., Tanir, M. & Akyildiz, S. (1999). Serum and peritoneal fluid levels of IGF I and II and insulin-like growth binding protein-3 in endometriosis, *J Reprod Med,* Vol. 44, No. 5, (May 1999), pp. 450–454, ISSN 0024-7758

Huber, A., Keck, C.C., Hefler, L.A., Schneeberger, C., Huber, J.C., Bentz, E.K. & Tempfer, C.B. (2005). Ten estrogen-related polymorphisms and endometriosis: a study of multiple gene-gene interactions, *Obst Gynecol,* Vol. 106, No. 5, (November 2005), pp. 1025-1031, ISSN 0029-7844

Illera, J.C., Silvan, G., Illera, M.J., Munro, C.J., Lessey, B.A. & Illera, M. (2001). Measurement of serum and peritoneal fluid LH concentrations as a diagnostic tool for human endometriosis, *Reproduction,* Vol. 121, No. 5, (May 2001), pp. 761–769, ISSN 1470-1626

Iwabe, T., Harada, T., Sakamoto, Y., Iba, Y., Horie, S., Mitsunari, M. & Terakawa, N. (2003). Gonadotropin-releasing hormone agonist treatment reduced serum interleukin-6 concentrations in patients with ovarian endometriomas, *Fertil Steril,* Vol. 80, No. 2, (August 2003), pp. 300-304, ISSN 0015-0282

Kawasaki, H., Onuki, R., Suyama, E. & Taira, K. (2002). Identification of genes that function in the TNFα-mediated apoptotic pathway using randomized hybrid ribozyme libraries, *Nat Biotechnol,* Vol. 20, No. 4, (April 2002), pp. 376-80, ISSN 1087-0156

Kitawaki, J., Kado, N., Ishihara, H., Koshiba, H., Kitaoka, Y. & Honjo, H. (2002). Endometriosis: the patophysiology as an estrogen-dependent disease, *J Steroid Biology,* Vol. 83, No. 1-5, (December 2002), pp. 149-155, ISSN 0960-0760

Konno, R., Yamakawa, H., Utsunomiya, H., Ito, K., Sato, S. & Yajima, A. (2000). Expression of survivin and Bcl-2 in the normal human endometrium, *Mol Hum Reprod,* Vol. 6, No. 6, (June 2000), pp. 529-534, ISSN 1360-9947

Lebovic, D.I., Mueller, M.D. & Taylor, R.N. (2001). Immunobiology of endometriosis *Fertil Steril,* Vol. 75, No. 1, (January 2001), pp. 1-10, ISSN 0015-0282

Leng, J., Lang, J., Zhao, D. & Liu, D. (2002). Serum levels of soluble intercellular molecule 1 (sICAM-1) in endometriosis, *Zhonghua Yi Xue Za Zhi*, Vol. 82, No. 3, (February 2002), pp. 189–190, ISSN 0376-2491

Matalliotakis, I.M., Goumenou, A.G., Koumantakis, G.E., Athanassakis, I., Dionyssopoulou, E., Neonaki, M.A. & Vassiliadis, S. (2003). Expression of serum human leukocyte antigen and growth factor levels in a Greek family with familial endometriosis, *J Soc Gynecol Investig*, Vol. 10, No. 2, (February 2002), pp. 118–121, ISSN 1071-5576

Matalliotakis, I.M., Goumenou, A.G., Koumantakis, G.E., Neonaki, M.A., Koumantakis, G.E., Dionyssopoulou, E., Athanassakis, I. & Vassiliadis, S. (2003). Serum concentrations of growth factors in women with and without endometriosis: the action of anti-endometriosis medicines, *Int Immunopharmacol*, Vol. 3, No. 1, (January 2003), pp. 81–89, ISSN 1567-5769

Mhawech, P., Kinkel, K., Vlastos, G. & Pelte, M.F. (2001). Ovarian carcinomas in endometriosis: an immunohistochemical and comparative genomic hybridization study, *Int J Gynecol Pathol*, Vol. 21, No. 4 (October 2001), pp. 401-406, ISSN 0277-1691

Nothnick, W.B. (2001). Treating endometriosis as an autoimmune disease, *Fertil Steril*, Vol. 76, No. 2, (August 2001), pp. 223–231, ISSN 0015-0282

Rier, S. & Foster, W.G. (2003). Environmental dioxins and endometriosis, *Sem Reprod Med*, Vol. 21, No. 2, (May 2003), pp. 145-154, ISSN 1526-8004

Sillem, M., Prifti, S., Koch, A., Neher, M., Jauckus, J. & Runnebaum, B. (2001). Regulation of matrix metalloproteinases and their inhibitors in uterine endometrial cells of patients with and without endometriosis, *Eur J Obstet Gynecol Reprod Biol*, Vol. 95, No. 2, (April 2001), pp. 167–174, ISSN 0301-2115

Somigliana, E., Viganò, P., Candiani, M., Felicetta, I., Di Blasio, A.M. & Vignali, M. (2003). Use of serum-soluble intercellular adhesion molecule-1 as a new marker of endometriosis, *Fertil Steril*, Vol. 77, No. 5, (May 2003), pp. 1028–1031, ISSN 0015-0282

Tanaka, T., Utsunomiya, T., Bai, T., Nakajima, S. & Umesaki, N. (2003). Leptin inhibits decidualization and enhances cell viability of normal human endometrial stromal cells, *Int J Mol Med*, Vol. 12, No. 1, (July 2003), pp. 95–98, ISSN 1107-3756

Taylor, R.N., Lundeen, S.G. & Giudice, L,C. (2002). Emerging role of genomics in endometriosis research, *Fertil Steril*, Vol. 78, No. 4, (October 2002), pp. 694-698, ISSN 0015-0282

Vietri, M.T., Molinari, A.M., Iannella, I., Cioffi, M., Bontempo, P., Ardovino, M., Scaffa, C., Colacurci, N. & Cobellis, L. (2007). Arg72Pro p53 polymorphism in Italian women: no association with endometriosis, *Fertil Steril*, Vol. 88, No. 5, (November 2007), pp. 1468-1469, ISSN 0015-0282

Vietri, M.T., Cioffi, M., Sessa, M., Simeone, S., Bontempo, P., Trabucco, E., Ardovino, M., Colacurci, N., Molinari, A.M. & Cobellis, L. (2009). CYP17 and CYP19 gene polymorphisms in women affected with endometriosis, *Fertil Steril*, Vol. 92, No. 5, (November 2009), pp. 1532-1535, ISSN 0015-0282

Viganò, P., Somigliana, E., Matrone, R., Dubini, A., Barron, C., Vignali, M. & di Blasio, A.M. (2002). Serum leptin concentrations in endometriosis, *J Clin Endocrinol Metabol*, Vol. 87, No. 3, (March 2002), pp. 1085–1087, ISSN 0021-972X

Wieser, F., Fabjani, G., Tempfer, C., Schneeberger, C., Sator, M., Huber, J. & Wenzi R. (2003). Analysis of an interleukin-6 gene promoter polymorphism in women with endometriosis by pyrosequencing, *J Soc Gynecol Investig,* Vol. 10, No. 1, (January 2003), pp. 32–36, ISSN 1071-5576

Zong, LL., Li, Y.L. & Ha, X.Q. (2003). Determination of HGF concentration in serum and peritoneal fluid in women with endometriosis, *Di Yi Jun Yi Da Xue Xue Bao,* Vol. 23, No. 8, pp. (August 2003), 757–760, ISSN 1000-2588

9

Pelvic Endometriosis: A MR Pictorial Review

Rosario Francesco Grasso, Riccardo Del Vescovo,
Roberto Luigi Cazzato and Bruno Beomonte Zobel
Department of Radiology, Campus Bio-Medico University of Rome,
Italy

1. Introduction

Endometriosis is one of the most common benign gynaecological conditions. It is defined as the presence of ectopic endometrial glands and stroma outside the uterus. The ectopic endometrium responds to hormonal stimulation with a cyclic hemorrhage, resulting in a complex spectrum of symptoms.

Pain is the cardinal symptom of endometriosis, even though patients may experience several different types of pain, such as dysmenorrhea, deep dyspareunia, discomfort during defecation or while urinating, according to the anatomic location of this disorder. Endometriotic implants, pelvic adhesions and ovarian endometriomas are commonly associated with chronic pelvic pain. Haemorrhage into an endometrioma may result in acute pain. Infertility is another commonly associated complaint.

The exact prevalence of endometriosis is not well defined, as the diagnostic gold standard is represented by laparoscopy or laparotomy. It is estimated about 5-10%, including both symptomatic and asymptomatic women. Nulliparous women and women reporting short and heavy menstrual cycles are at increased risk [1]; these epidemiological findings support the metastatic implantation from retrograde menstruation hypothesis. Other theories include the metaplastic differentiation of serosal surfaces or müllerian remnant tissue, and the induction of undifferentiated mesenchyme to form endometriotic tissue due to released substances from the shed endometrium (induction theory) [2].

The most common locations of endometriosis are the ovaries and the pelvic peritoneum, followed in order of decreasing frequency by deep lesions of the pelvic subperitoneal space, the intestinal system and the urinary system. Deep pelvic endometriosis is a pathologically distinct entity: deep endometriotic lesions penetrate under the surface of peritoneum (infiltration > 5mm) and are tipically found in the uterosacral ligaments, rectum, rectovaginal septum, vagina or bladder, and induce a fibromuscolar hyperplasia that surrounds endometriosis foci [3].

The diagnosis of endometriosis still remains a challenge for clinicians, resulting from similarities in clinical symptoms to other benign or malignant gynaecological diseases.

Laparoscopy is the standard of reference in the diagnosis of endometriosis; histological analysis of biopsy specimens should confirm the diagnosis, even if it is not necessary.

On the other hand, laparoscopy is also required for staging the disease. The most widely used staging system is the 1985 Revised Classification of Endometriosis published by the

American Fertility Society [4]. The rAFS score takes into account the presence of ovarian and peritoneal implants (subdivided into superficial or deep), the severity of the adhesions and the presence or not of a complete posterior cul-de-sac obliteration (i.e. frozen pelvis). The rAFS staging system has shown poor correlation to the clinical severity of the disease, so requiring further refinement. Meanwhile a new staging system called ENZIAN score has been recently developed [5]; it is focused on the deep pelvic endometriosis that is the most severe form of the disease.

The clinical value of this staging system and its correlation to the reproductive prognosis of endometriosis patients should be assessed.

Therapeutic options are observation, medical treatment, surgery or a combination strategy.

The most widely used medical therapy of endometriosis includes oral contraceptives, androgenic agents, progestins, and gonadotropin releasing hormone (GnRH) analogs. The choice of a surgical option depends upon the severity of the disease. Surgery is the main therapeutic option in patients with deep pelvic endometriosis. Anterior cul-de-sac endometriosis involving the bladder can be treated with laparoscopic surgery. Preoperative staging of disease is necessary because in certain cases surgery should be performed by standard laparotomy (bladder endometriosis associated with bowel involvement). Treatment of posterior cul-de-sac endometriosis can be achieved with laparoscopy, but a vaginal or a laparotomic approach is needed when vaginal or severe bowel disease, respectively are present.

2. Pathologic features of endometriosis

The most common site of involvement is the ovary, but virtually all pelvic organs can be affected by the disease.

Ovarian endometriosis includes a superficial form, which appears as small punctuate foci measuring no more than 5 mm, and a 'deep' one; in the latter case the typical aspect is that of the "chocolate cyst" or "endometrioma". Chocolate cysts typically have thick, fibrotic walls, a dark-brown, viscous content and their diameter rarely exceed 15 cm.

Aspect of endometriotic peritoneal implants ranges from punctuate foci to small stellar patches; according to the age of the lesion and the amount of pigment, they could appear white, yellow, red, blue or brown (**Fig. 1**).

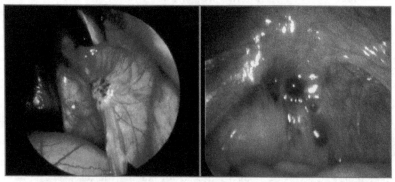

Fig. 1. Endometriotic nodules as they are seen in laparoscopy

When the peritoneal lesion invades the subserosal layers it progressively leads to extensive fibrosis, wall thickening of the pelvic organs, nodule formation and distortion of the normal pelvic anatomy due to a fibrous retraction; the most severe form is the so called "frozen pelvis", that consists of a huge amount of tissue involving the retro-uterine excavation and causing an extensive infiltration of the posterior pelvis (torus uteri, uterosacral ligaments, vaginal and rectal wall).

Microscopic appearance of endometriosis is composed of endometrial glands, stroma and occasionally histiocytes, due to an inflammatory response caused by cyclic hemorrhages within the implant. In rare cases endometriosis may lack glands (stromal endometriosis) [6].

3. Radiologic evaluation of endometriosis

Radiologists are often involved in the diagnosis and pre-operative assessment of the disease: an accurate pre-operative evaluation of the endometrial implants (location, size and depth of penetration) could help the surgeon to perform a radical surgical excision in cases in which severe fibrosis and adhesions hide deep lesions and impede laparoscopic evaluation.

Imaging methods that are used in the daily practice to diagnose endometriosis are ecotomografy, especially Transvaginal Ultrasound (TVUS) and Magnetic Resonance Imaging (MRI).

TVUS provides high resolution images of the pelvic organs, providing reliable information in patients with both acute and chronic pelvic pain [7].

The classic endometrioma on TVUS appears as an area of low and homogenous echoes.

TVUS has been reported to be the best method for discriminating between endometriotic and non-endometriotic cysts, with a sensitivity of 83% and a false positive rate of 7%. The addition of CA-125 evaluation does not improve the diagnostic accuracy of TVUS, thus indicating TVUS alone to be the least expensive instrument for identifying the presence of endometriomas [8,9].

The role of TVUS for the assessment of deep pelvic endometriosis has been recently reported, with conflicting results. TVUS is apparently more accurate than Rectal Endoscopic Ultrasound (RES) for predicting deep pelvic endometriosis in specific locations and should be the first line imaging method in this setting [10]. RES appears to be the best technique for evaluating the depth of bowel infiltration by endometriosis [11].

The role of MRI in the diagnosis of endometriosis has increased after 1987, when Nishimura et al. [12] demonstrated the value of this imaging method in the diagnosis of endometriomas. Then the use of MRI for the evaluation of deep endometriosis was proposed by Siegelman et al. [13], who studied its role in analysing solid pelvic masses. More recently other investigators [14] showed the promising results of MRI for the specific evaluation of deep endometriosis.

Also dynamic MR imaging has been tested for this purpose, showing a good accuracy in the differential diagnosis of nodular endometriosis from other pathologic conditions of abdominal wall and pelvis [15].

4. MRI technique

In our experience, MRI studies are performed with a 1.5 T magnet (Magnetom Symphony; Siemens Erlangen, Germany) and a surface phased-array coil. Patient preparation requires intravenous injection of an antispasmodic drug prior to study in order to reduce artefacts from bowel motion.

On the basis of the characteristics of our system, the standard imaging protocol includes a coronal T2-weighted HASTE sequence (half-Fourier single shot turbo spin echo: TR 700 ; TE 89; section thickness 6.0 mm; field of view 350x450 mm; matrix 320; time of acquisition 21 s), transverse T1-weighted turbo spin echo sequences from the iliac crest to the pubic sinfisis (TR 771; TE 9.7; section thickness 4.0 mm; field of view 400 x 219 mm; matrix 512x512; time of acquisition 2:46), transverse, sagittal and coronal T2-weighted turbo spin echo sequences. These sequences allow an initial complete analysis of the pelvic region and a preliminary evaluation of endometriotic lesions, which appear as hyperintense lesions in T1-weighted sequences and mildly hypointense or hyperintense in T2 weighted sequences. The FLASH T1-weighted sequences with fat suppression in transverse, coronal and sagittal plane (Fast Low-Angle Shot 2D: TR 357; TE 4.76; FA 70°; section thikness 4.5 mm; field of view 300x300 mm; matrix 256x256; time of acquisition 1:31) (T1 flash 2d fat sat) are performed to evaluate adnexal masses because they allow a distinction between a fatty content lesion (for example a teratoma, which appear hypointense in fat-suppressed T1 weighted sequences) and endometriomal cyst (that exhibits a typical hyperintense signal in such sequences). Fat-suppressed MRI is also useful in enhancing the contrast between hemorrhagic implants and normal tissue.

Contrast-enhanced FLASH T1-weighted sequences (gadolinium Gd-DTPA 0.1 mmol/kg is administrated intravenously) are performed in selected cases, expecially when a mural nodule within a hyperintense endometrioma is observed. Finally, the contrast agent is administrated when the initial images carry the suspicion of ureteral infiltration. In such cases we perform FLASH 3D T1 weighted sequences in the coronal plane with MIP recostruction of 1 mm (MR Urography) (TR: 2.96; TE 1.21; section thickness 1.40 mm; field of view 350x490 mm; matrix 384; time of acquisition 20 sec).

5. Spectrum of MRI findings

The diagnosis of endometriosis by means of MRI is based on the combination of two aspects: presence abdominal areas with morphologic and signal intensity abnormalities. Endometriotic lesions appear hyperintense on T1-weighted images and mildly hypointense or hyperintense on T2-weighted images (**Fig. 2A, B**). Gradual variation of signal intensity on T2-weighted images has been described as the "shading" sign (**Fig. 2A**) and it is due to chronic bleeding with accumulation of high concentration of iron and protein in the endometrioma.

Fat saturation allows differentiation between hemorrhagic (endometriomas) and fatty (dermoid cyst) content of cystic lesions (**Fig. 3**). Moreover, it increases detection of small implants.

Use of contrast-enhanced imaging is required to identify solid enhancing nodules within endometriotic cysts when malignant transformation is suspected or to define the extent of inflammation associated with endometriosis.

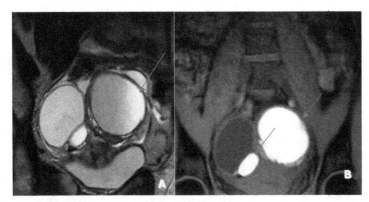

Fig. 2. Endometriotic lesions appear mildly hypointense or hyperintense on T2-weighted images (A) and hyperintense on T1-weighted images (arrows in B). Gradual variation of signal intensity on T2-weighted images has been described as "shading" sign and is due to chronic bleeding with accumulation of high concentration of iron and protein in endometriomas (arrows in A).

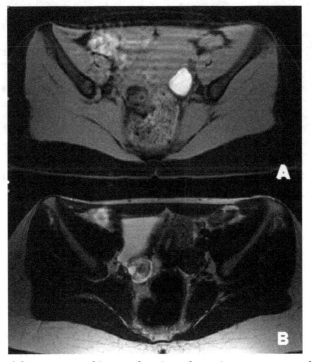

Fig. 3. T1-weighted-fat-suppressed image showing a hyperintense mass on the left ovary and a disomogenous hypointense mass on the right one (A). On T2-weighted sequence (B) the left mass appear hypointense. The left mass proved to be an endometrioma with recent hemorrhage; on the contrary, owing to its appeareance on fat-suppressed sequence, the right mass proved to be a dermoid syst.

5.1 Ovarian endometriosis

Adnexal localization is the most common clinical setting of endometriosis.

TVUS remains the first diagnostic method in the evaluation of the ovary, generally reserving MRI as a tool for resolving cases in which there is some doubt.

At MRI, a large endometrioma (>1 cm in diameter) appears as a homogeneously hyperintense mass on T1 weighted MR images and show a low signal intensity on T2 weighted MR images with areas of high signal intensity. The 'shading' sign is used to differentiate endometriomas from functional hemorrhagic cysts that do not show it, which usually disappears at subsequent MRI examinations.

Another diagnostic criteria for a definitive diagnosis of endometriomas is the presence of multiple T1 hyperintense cysts regardless of their T2 signal intensity [16].

Endometriomas are often bilateral (more than 50% of cases), multilocular or associated with interovarian adhesions; in the last case a typical MRI pattern called "kissing ovaries" could be noted (**Fig. 4**).

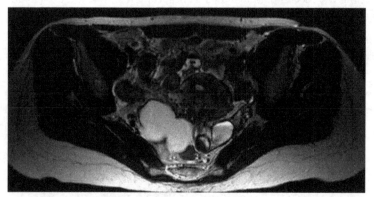

Fig. 4. T2-weighted image acquired on the transverse plane, showing hyperintense bilateral endometrioma masses on the ovaries that are closed up due to interovarian adhesions (Kissing ovaries).

Fat suppression is mandatory to differentiate endometriomas from cystic teratomas.

5.2 'Deep endometriosis'

Deep endometriotic lesions are classified according to the anatomic location in the anterior compartment (bladder) or in the posterior compartment (uterosacral ligament, vagina and bowel).

Multifocality is a major characteristic of deep endometriosis, thus requiring in some cases different surgical procedures (laparoscopy and/or laparotomy) to obtain a complete exeresis and a functional improvement.

5.3 Endometriosis of the bladder

Localization of disease in the bladder is estimated in < 1% of patients.

Uterus is usually anteflexed and the anterior cul-de-sac is obliterated due to extensive adhesions. The patient often complain pain, especially while urinating.

Two types of bladder endometriosis have been recognised. One develops exclusively after cesarean section and is considered to result from iatrogenic implantation of decidua. The other, a primary form, is found in women who have not previously undergone surgery on the uterus. Various hypotheses have been proposed to explain the pathogenesis in the latter case. Microscopically, the typical pattern is a focus of endometriosis scattered in the bladder wall. The main feature is the paucity of endometrial-type stroma [17].

MRI is reliable for the diagnosis of bladder endometriosis. Endocavitary coil MRI is reliable for establishing the depth of the lesions penetrating into the bladder wall [18].

On MRI images, bladder endometriosis can be diagnosed as a localized or diffuse bladder wall thickening, or as focal signal intensity abnormality. T2 and T1 weighted images can show a nodular hypointense mass usually located on the anterior upper or posterior bladder wall (**Fig. 5**).

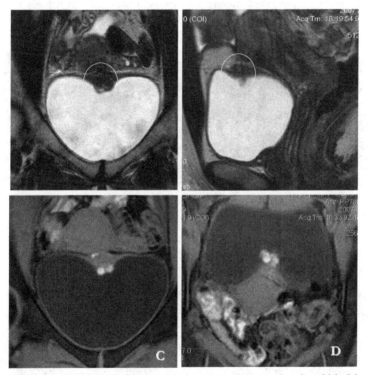

Fig. 5. Coronal (A) and sagittal (B) T2-weighted images showing localized bladder wall thickening in the anterior upper bladder wall (blue circles). On fat suppressed T1-weighted coronal (C) and axial (D) images some high signal intensity intra-lesion spots indicating recent haemorrage.

On fat suppressed T1-weighted FLASH 2d images, some high signal intensity intralesional spots are present in some cases.

5.4 Endometriosis of the uterosacral ligaments (USLs)

USLs are one of the most common targets of pelvic endometriosis, which is diagnosed more frequently in a clinical than in a surgical setting. USLs extend over a mean cranio-caudal distance of 21±8 mm. Three regions of origin have been found: cervix alone, vagina alone, cervix and vagina. Insertion points are the piriformis muscle, the sciatic foramen and the ischial spine [19].

This affliction often elicits pelvic pain, dyspareunia and painful bowel movement.

Women with endometriosis in this site present thick USLs due to endometriotic nodules and subsequently, fibrosis is responsible for cul-de-sac obliteration.

TVUS may provide quantitative information to manage patients with USLs endometriosis [20].

At MRI, involvement of USLs by endometriosis is diagnosed when the ligament appears thickened or shows irregular margins (**Fig. 6**) compared with the margins of the controlateral ligament. T2-weighted images identify all lesions as iso- or hypointense to myometrium, while T1-weighted images are less sensitive due to lesions isointensity to myometrium. The proximal portion of the ligament typically presents with asymmetric nodular thickening.

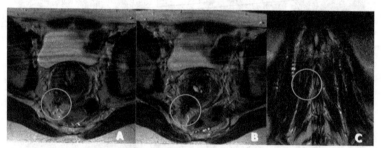

Fig. 6. Axial (A and B) and coronal (C) T2-weighted images showing irregular thickening of the right Utero-Sacral ligaments (blue circles). On the same image there is infiltration of the rectal serosa (blue circle).

Fat-suppressed T1-weighted images sometimes demonstrate hyperintense spots that correlate with hemorrhagic endometrial implants on the ligament (**Fig. 7**).

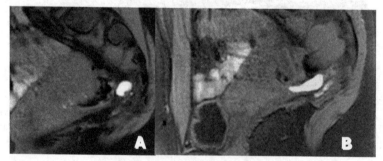

Fig. 7. Fat-suppressed T1-weighted images demonstrate hyperintense spots that correlate with hemorrhagic endometrial implants on the ligament (A, B).

In patients with USLs involvement adhesions could often develop thus, providing posterior displacement of the uterus and ovaries, angulation of bowel loops, elevation of the posterior vaginal fornix, and loculated fluid collections [21]. At MRI, adhesions are detected when low signal intensity is found within the ligaments.

5.5 Endometriosis of the vagina

Endometriosis of the vagina includes lesions infiltrating the anterior rectovaginal pouch, posterior vaginal fornix and retroperitoneal area between the anterior rectovaginal pouch and posterior vaginal fornix.

Patients tipycally refer dyspareunia.

MRI represents the ideal complement to physical examination and TVUS in order to predict lesion extension upward and posteriorly. Sometimes, the use of a water enema is used to predict the extension of the lesion toward the rectum.

In patients with vaginal endometriosis axial and sagittal T2-weighted Turbo Spin Echo images usually show hypointense nodules. Anterior attraction of the rectum toward the torus uteri and asymmetric thickening of the rectal wall are associated to rectal wall infiltration. Determining the depth of infiltration of the rectal wall allows the gynaecologist to discuss the surgical approach (nodulectomy vs bowel resection) with the colorectal surgeon. The use of the endorectal coil optimizes the finding of MRI [22].

T1-weighted images with fat suppression could demonstrate T1 isointensity of the nodule and some small hyperintense foci, suspected for micro-haemorrhages (**Fig. 8 A**).

Most patients with vaginal involvement also demonstrate obliteration of the retrouterine excavation (**Fig. 8 B, C**); in such cases the extension of the pelvic focus may lead to ureteral infiltration and ureterohydronephrosis.

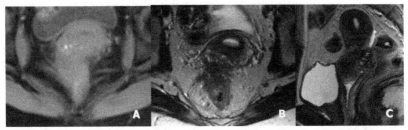

Fig. 8. T1-weighted image with fat suppression demonstrates isointensity of the nodule and some small hyperintense foci, suspected for micro-haemorrhages (A). Axial (B) and sagittal (C) T2-weighted image show obliteration of retrouterine escavation by an hypointense nodule, with anterior attraction of the rectum toward the torus uteri and asymmetric thickening of the rectal wall.

5.6 Endometriosis of the bowel

Rectosigmoid endometriosis represents 70% of cases of intestinal endometriosis.

Clinical symptoms of patients with endometriosis of the recto-sigmoid colon are manifested as crampy pain, flatulence, painful tenesmus, constipation, diarrhoea and bowel obstruction.

Among patients with rectosigmoid endometriosis also dyspareunia is another common symptom. Endometriosis less frequently affects appendix, cecum and distal ileum.

The implants are usually serosal but they can erode through the subserosal layers and cause a fibromuscular hyperplasia of the muscularis propria. Due to the normal appearance of the mucosa in most patients with bowel endometriosis, diagnosis by colonoscopy is often false negative. The appearance of gastrointestinal implants on double-contrast barium enema images is characterized in most cases by a puckering or a crenulated appearance of the affected wall; when the lesion causes a circumferential narrowing of the rectosigmoid colon the differential diagnosis with a primary colon carcinoma is difficult.

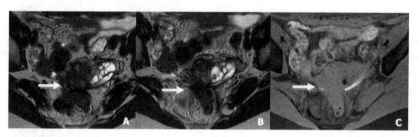

Fig. 9. Diagnostic criteria of bowel invasion at MRI are: colorectal wall thickening with traction of the rectum toward the torus uteri (A, B, C).

At MRI, bowel lesions show a signal intensity similar to fibromuscular tissue (hypointense), with occasional hyperintense foci of T1- and T2- weighted images. An asymmetric thickening of the lower surface of the sigmoid wall or a colorectal wall thickening with attraction of the rectum toward the torus uteri is a common sign (**Fig. 9**).

According to Roy C *et al* [23], the use of the contrast media helps in reaching the diagnosis of an invasion inside the muscular layer of the intestinal wall. In such cases a thin bright layer on T2-weighted images together with post-contrast enhancement on fat-suppressed T1-weighted images and obliteration of fatty tissue plane between the nodule and the intestinal wall, represents the diagnostic clue of muscular layers involvement. Combined pelvic-phased array and endovaginal coils improve the diagnostic power in the detection of intestinal wall invasion, when compared to phased array alone.

5.7 Malignant transformation

A limited number of endometriosis patients (<5%) will develop ovarian cancer.

Women with endometriosis-associated cancer are typically pre-menopausal, have high incidence of endometrioid and clear cell histologies, and have early stage disease [24].

The association between endometriosis and intra-peritoneal cancer still remains unclear. Probably, women with endometriosis are more susceptible to malignant transformation because of a deficit in their immune system that enables the endometriosis to flourish. Also estrogen may play a role, so endometriosis should be closely monitored in women in the reproductive age [25].

The typical morphologic appearance of an endometriosis-associated carcinoma is that of a unilateral large cystic mass containing hemorrhagic fluid and mural nodules. Signal intensity is low on T1-weighted images and variable on T2-weighted images. Contrast enhancement of a mural nodule at fat-suppressed T1-weighted sequences is the most important finding for a diagnosis of malignant shift. The "shading" sign within the cystic mass is rarely observed on T2-weighted images because of the diluition of the hemorrhagic fluid caused by tumor secretions. Accordingly, disappearance of the "shading" sign within the mass on T2-weighted images is a diagnostic clue to its malignancy [26].

6. Conclusions

MRI is progressively becoming a widely employed technique in the diagnosis and preoperative staging of endometriosis. It should be performed in selected patients according to the results of TVUS and the severity of symptoms. This imaging method has the advantage to cover the entire pelvis thus, helping the surgeon to achieve a complete resection and prevent post-surgical recurrence.

7. References

[1] Missmer SA & Cramer DW. The epidemiology of endometriosis. Obstetrics and Gynecology Clinics of North America 2003 ; 30 : 1-19

[2] Olive DL, Schwartz LB. Endometriosis. N Engl J Med 1993; 328:1759–1769

[3] Chapron C, Fauconnier A, Vieira M, Barakat H, Dousset B, Pansini V, Vacher-Lavenu MC, Dubuisson J.B.. Anatomical Distribution of deeply infiltrating endometriosis : surgical implications and proposition for a classification. Hum Reprod 2003; 18:157-161.

[4] Revised American fertility Society classification of endometriosis: 1985. Fertil Steril 1985; 43: 351-352.

[5] Tuttlies F. et al. ENZIAN-Score, eine Klassifikation der tief infiltrierenden Endometriose: Zentralbl Gynacol 2005; 127: 275-282.

[6] Clement PB. Diseases of the peritoneum. In: Kurman RJ, ed. Blaustein's pathology of the female genital tract. 4th ed New York, NY: Springer-Verlag, 1994; 660-680.

[7] Okaro E, Valentin L. The role of ultrasound in the management of women with acute and chronic pelvic pain. Best Practice and Research Clinical Obstetrics and Gynaecology 2004, Vol 18 No 1 1 pp 105-123.

[8] Mais V, Guerriero S, Ajossa S, Angiolucci M, Paoletti AM, Melis GB. The efficiency of transvaginal ultrasonography in the diagnosis of endometrioma. Fertil and Steril 1993, 60:776-780.

[9] Guerriero S, Mais V, Ajossa S, Paoletti AM, Angiolucci M, Melis GB. Transvaginal ultrasonography combined with CA-125 plasma levels in the diagnosis of endometrioma. Fertil and Steril 1996, 65:293-298.

[10] Bazot M., Malzy P., Cortez A., Roseau G., Amouyal P., Darai E. Accuracy of transvaginale sonosgraphy and rectal endoscopic sonography in the diagnosis of deep infiltrating endometriosis. Ultrasound Obstet Gynecol 2007; 30:994-1001.

[11] Chapron C, Vieira M., Chopin N, Balleyguier C, Barakat H, Dumontier I, Roseau G, Fauconnier A, Foulot H, Dousset B. Accuracy of rectal endoscopic ultrasonography and magnetic resonance imaging in the diagnosis of rectal involvement for patients presenting with deeply infiltrating endometriosis. Ultrasound Obstet Gynecol 2004; 24:175-179.

[12] Nishimura K, Togashi K, Itoh K, Fujisawa I, Noma S, Kawamura Y, Nakano Y, Itoh H, Torizuka K, Ozasa H. Endometrial cysts of the ovary: MR imaging. Radiology. 1987 Feb;162(2):315-8.

[13] Siegelman ES, Outwater E, Wang T, Mitchell DG. Solid pelvic masses caused by endometriosis: MR imaging features. AJR Am J Roentgenol. 1994 Aug;163(2):357-61.

[14] Bazot M, Darai E, Hourani R, Thomassin I, Cortez A, Uzan S, Buy JN. Deep pelvic endometriosis: MR imaging for diagnosis and prediction of extension of disease. Radiology. 2004 Aug;232(2):379-89

[15] Onbas O, Kantarci M, Alper F, Kumtepe Y, Durur I, Ingec M, Gursan N, Okur A. Nodular endoimetriosis: dynamic MR imaging. Abdominal Imaging 2007, 32: 451-456.

[16] Togashi K, Nishimura K, Kimura I et al . Endometrial cysts: diagnosis with MR imaging. Radiology 1991. 180: 73-78.

[17] Fedele L, Piazzola E, Raffaelli R, Bianchi S. Bladder endometriosis: deep infiltrating endometriosis or adenomyosis?. Fertil and Steril. 1998; 69: 972-974.

[18] Halleguier C, Chapron C, Dubuisson J B, Kinkel K, Fauconnier A, Vieira M et al.. Comparison of Magnetic Resonance Imaging and Transvaginal Ultrasonography in diagnosing bladder endometriosis. The journal of the American Association of Gynecologic Laparoscopy 2002; 9 (1) 15-23.

[19] Umek W H, Morgan D M, Ashton-Miller J A, DeLancey J O L. Quantitative analysis of uterosacral ligament origin and insertion points by magnetic resonance imaging. The American College of Obstetricians and Gynecologists. 2004; vol 103, no. 3, 447-451.

[20] Ohba T, Mizutani H, Maeda T, Matsuura K, Okamura H. Evaluation of endometriosis in uterosacral ligaments by transrectal ultrasonography. Human Reproduction 1996; vol 11 no.9 2014-17.

[21] Zawin M, McCarthy S, Scoutt L, Comite F. Endometriosis: appearance and detection at MR imaging. Radiology 1989; 171:693–696

[22] Kinkel K, Chapron C, Balleyguier C, Fritel X, Dubuisson JB, Moreau JF. Magnetic resonance imaging characteristics of deep endometriosis. Hum Reprod. 1999 Apr;14(4):1080-6.

[23] Roy C, Balzan C, Thoma V, Sauer B, wattiez A, Leroy J. Efficiency of MR imaging to orientate surgical treatment of posterior deep pelvic endometriosis. Abdom Imaging 2008; XX:1-9.

[24] S. C. Modessitt, G. Tortolero-Luna, J. B. Robinson. D.M. Gerhenson, J.K. Wolf Ovarian and Extraovarian-Associated Cancer The American College of Obstetricians and Gynecologists Vol. 100, No. 4, October 2002 788- 794

[25] Mc Meekin DS, Burger RA, Manetta A, Di Saia P, Barman ML. Endometrioid adenocarcinoma of the ovary and its relationship to endometriosis. Gynecol Oncol. 1995; 59:81-86

[26] M Takeuchi, K Matsuzaki, H. Uehara, H. Nishitani. Malignant transformation of Pelvic Endometriosis: MR Imaging findings and pathologic correlation. Radiographics 2006; 26:407-417

10

Imaging Tools for Endometriosis: Role of Ultrasound, MRI and Other Imaging Modalities in Diagnosis and Planning Intervention

Shalini Jain Bagaria[1], Darshana D. Rasalkar[2] and Bhawan K. Paunipagar[2]
[1]Department of Obstetrics & Gynecology, UCMS & GTB Hospital, Dilshad Garden,
[2]Department of Imaging and Interventional Radiology,
The Chinese University of Hong Kong, Prince of Wales Hospital,
Hong Kong

1. Introduction

Endometriosis is the presence of endometrial glands as well as stroma at the locations outside uterus. It affects up to 10% of women. Grossly there are three forms of the disease, namely a) superficial endometrial implants, b) ovarian endometriomas or endometriotic cysts, and c) deep infiltrating endometriosis. All the three forms depict varied manifestation of a single disease and require a careful pre operative work up to know the extent and distribution of the disease precisely as it is critical to frame the plan of management.

The superficial implants are typically 2-3 mm in size rooted in the serosal tissue of the peritoneum. They initially appear as red highly vascular lesions. Later, repeated haemorrhage and inflammation triggers fibrosis and haemosiderin deposition in them causing raised powder burn lesions. It is hard to find such lesions by USG or MRI. Traditional method of diagnostic endoscopy still remains the golden standard of reference to diagnose and stage this form of disease.

Endometriomas of the ovary or chocolate cysts of the ovary contain degraded blood products. The dark and gelatinous material in them is surrounded by fibrous wall of variable thickness. Endomeriotic cysts are often bilateral and multiple. Both the USG and MRI play key role in its evaluation.

The deep infiltrating endometriosis (DIE) is defined as the implant penetrating into the retroperitoneal space or the wall of the pelvic organs to the depth of at least 5mm. (Knoninckx et al). They usually appear as solid nodules. These types of lesions permeate deep into the surrounding fibromuscular tissues and induce smooth muscle proliferation and fibrous reaction effecting development of solid nodules. In case of visceral involvement, they can infiltrate into the muscle layer from the serosal layer. The resulting smooth muscle proliferation can lead to stricture formation and later obstruction.

2. Natural history of the disease

The natural history of the symptomatic disease is uncertain. The lesions may either continue to be same or may evolve further or may regress. Its malignant transformation is uncommon and its exact incidence is not known. This is diagnosed only if there is no evidence of metastasis from any primary sites and the surrounding tissue has presence of benign as well as the malignant endometrial tissue.

3. Locations

The disease most commonly affects the ovaries and the pelvic peritoneum. DIE classically affects the rectovaginal septum and the uterine ligaments (69.2%), the vagina (14.5%), the rectosigmoid bowel (9.9%), and the bladder and ureter (6.4%) in the order of frequency. Rarely lungs and CNS may be involved.

4. Diagnostic modalities for evaluation of endometriosis

The diagnosis of endometriosis is conventionally made by laparoscopy but over the time the imaging techniques have evolved to greatly facilitate the pre operative diagnosis. Further laparoscopy has limited role in visualizing atypical non pigmented extraperitoneal sites of involvement and the areas especially concealed by pelvic adhesions.

By and large ultrasound is the first preliminary investigation done to assess the pelvic disease in reproductive age group. Although it has limited role in detection of superficial implants, it is useful in the diagnosis and treatment of endometriomas. MRI provides a good alternative with high specificity and sensitivity for detecting deep infiltrating (DIE) endometriosis as well as endometriomas. The main drawback of MRI is again inability to detect small peritoneal infiltrates (< 3mm). Introduction of fat saturated T1 weighted image on MRI has consistently improved its accuracy in distinguishing between ovarian mass with lipids from endometriomas.

Computed tomography usually gives ill defined results, thus is not very helpful. Conventional investigations like barium enema or intravenous urography may prove useful in detection of visceral endometriosis. Their use however is limited in current practice due to excessive radiation dose.

Further sections of this chapter will first discuss the various imaging modalities in detail followed by the characteristic appearance of diverse typical and atypical forms of endometriosis.

4.1 Ultrasound

Ultrasound as discussed is usually the first investigation done in subject suspected of any pelvic disease. USG has the advantage of having good resolution, easy accessibility, less expensive, and is free of ionizing radiation. Three modes are available- transabdominal, transvaginal and endorectal scanning.

For transabdominal scanning 3-5 MHz convex probe is used. Full bladder is must for this technique in order to properly visualize the uterus and the ovaries. It is very useful in cases of suspected bladder involvement and abdominal wall endometriosis. Kidneys should be examined for hydronephrosis

Transvaginal scanning (TVS) is done with probe of high frequency 6-7.5MHz positioned in vagina. Full bladder is not a pre requisite for this mode of USG and procedure is well

Imaging Tools for Endometriosis: Role of Ultrasound, MRI and Other Imaging Modalities in Diagnosis and Planning Intervention

143

accepted by most of the patients. TVS has superior image quality and resolution as compared to TAS. Thus it has high sensitivity (92%) and specificity (99%) in detecting endometriomas. The typical ultrasound findings include a cystic mass with diffuse, low-level echoes (figure 1).

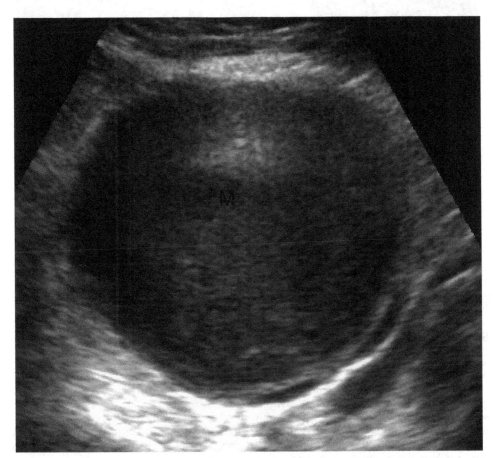

Fig. 1. Grey-scale Transvaginal ultrasound of an endometrioma(M). Note the characteristic diffuse, low-level echoes of the endometrioma giving a solid appearance

Depending on the age of the haemorrhage, the contents of the cyst, may vary in appearance. At times, an endometrioma may resemble a cystic-solid or entirely solid mass. Punctate echogenicities in the wall of endometriomas are less commonly seen but add specificity to the diagnosis. Endometriomas can be multilocular with internal thin or thick septations and thick irregular walls. Mild vascularity may be identified on color Doppler (figure 2). Color Doppler US shows no blood flow in the fine septations, whereas blood flow can often be detected in thick septations because of revascularization of chronic haematoma. Internal moving echos within endometrioma may reveal color signal.

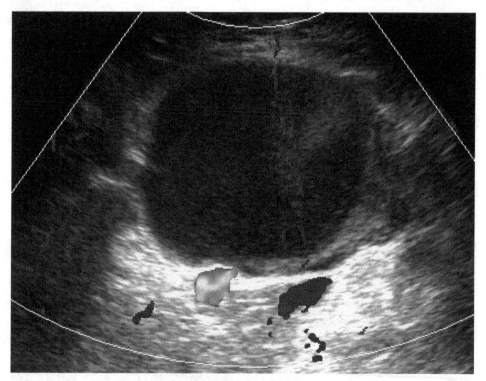

Fig. 2. Transvaginal ultrasound of an endometrioma color Doppler image showing mild peripheral vascularity. Internal color signals are likely related to moving internal echos.

Spectral Doppler reveal low-resistance waveforms which may not be helpful in differentiating endometriomas from other masses including malignancy.

Transrectal sonography uses biplane convex flexible rectal probe of 6.5MHz. The probe is flexible and can be advanced into the sigmoid colon to look for any signs of invasion by endometriosis. Patient preparation with rectal enema is required before endorectal sonography. The rectum and the surrounding area in the perimetry show five alternating hyper and hypoechoic layers respectively. The endometriotic deposits are visualized as triangular or round hypoechoic lesions on transrectal USG. It is superior to MRI with reported high sensitivity and specificity of 97% and 80%.

4.2 Magnetic resonance imaging

MRI is a non invasive intervention by which whole pelvis can be visualized in different planes. It can be very useful in patients in whom ultrasound findings are equivalent and in carefully selected high risk population. It is especially beneficial in identifying endometriomas, adhesions, superficial peritoneal implants and extraperitoneal lesions, particularly those in the rectovaginal space and uterosacral ligaments as well as in solid endometriotic nodules. In view of longer imaging times required for MRI, antiperistaltic medication to decrease the bowel movement can minimize motion related artifact and also enhances the visualization of the bowel involvement.

The signal intensity of MRI depends on the contents of the endometrial implants. The contents of these implants mainly include the proteins and degraded blood products, the ratio of which varies according to the stage of the haemorrhage and thus the variation in the signal intensity can be noted on MR images. The acute haemorrhage may give hypointense (dark) signal on the T1 and T2 weighted images. In contrast the lesions containing degraded blood products like methemoglobin, proteins and iron may be seen as hyperintense (bright) on T1 (figure 3) and hypointense (dark) on T2 weighted images(figure 4). Multiple high signal lesions, usually in the ovaries, on T1-weighted images, also are highly suggestive of endometriosis. The diagnostic MR imaging features of endometrioma include cystic mass with high signal intensity on T1-weighted images and loss of signal intensity on T2-weighted images. This phenomenon is referred to as "shading" as a result of high protein and iron concentration from recurrent hemorrhage in the endometrioma.

The advent of fat saturated T1 weighted technique has greatly enhanced the value of MRI in differentiating among endometriomas and lipid containing ovarian tumors like dermoid cysts. Use of contrast medium (Gadolinium) has not shown any advantage over plain MRI for the purpose but it may be useful when malignant lesion is suspected.

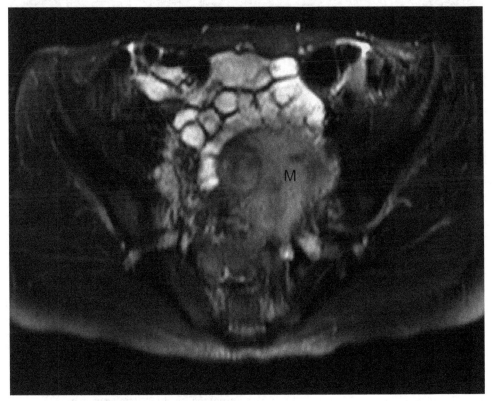

Fig. 3. Axial fat saturated T1Weighted image reveals T1 hyperintense lesions in the left ovary (M) suggestive a chocolate cyst/endrometrioma of the ovary.

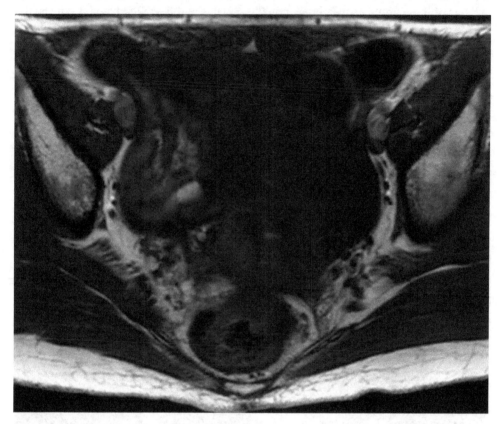

Fig. 4. Axial T2Weighted image showing the lesions are hypointense on T2W images.

The solid nodules of DIE appear as low intermediate signal on T1 weighted with punctuate areas of high signal and uniform low signals on T2 weighted images. The high signal zone is the consequence of foci of haemorrhage bounded by fibrous tissues. However it is difficult to identify superficial peritoneal implants on MRI.

Adhesions in the pelvis are one of the hallmarks of the disease. They appear as low signal areas of stranding. Adhesions are also suggested by the fixed retroverted uterus, angulated loops of bowel or displacement of the ovaries. Complications of endometriosis such as bowel implants and ureteral obstruction can often be detected on MRI.

It is now feasible to see the visceral deposits on MRI directly. Rather some studies claim MR imaging to be more specific than endorectal USG with sensitivity and specificity of 90-92% and 91 to 98% respectively (Gougoutas CA et al). MRI has valuable role in identification of nerve invasion (sciatic endometriosis) and abdominal wall lesions. The accuracy of MRI has been improved with the introduction of newer approach particularly endocavitary and phased array coils.

Role of MRI has been analyzed by various authors in the past. Stratton et al in a study reported 69% sensitivity and 75% specificity for detecting endometriosis confirmed on biopsy. MRI proposed diagnosis in nearly all patients with the severe form of the disease but by and large could recognize only small number of endometriotic areas as compared to surgery. Thus it is relatively less sensitive in determining the extent of the disease.

With this background in mind, the next section of the chapter will discuss in detail the features specific to different types of endometriosis on USG and MRI.

5. Different types of endometriosis

5.1 Superficial implants

Both USG and MRI has major limitation in diagnosing this type of endometriosis as already discussed. Endoscopy remains the standard practice to determine the extent of involvement by such lesions.

5.2 Endometriomas

Transvaginal sonography (TVS) is universally most frequently used imaging tool for evaluation of endometriomas. USG features of chocolate cysts are diverse. The classical appearance is that of a cystic structure with diffuse low level internal echoes and echogenic wall foci. The cyst may be unilocular or multilocular. It may contain thin or thick septa. Sometimes there may be wall nodularity. Wall nodularity if present requires further investigation to rule out malignancy. Imaging alone cannot exclude malignant neoplasm.

It is interesting to note that out of 20% of the endometriomas exhibiting wall nodularity, 35% had hyperechogenic wall foci (Patel et al). Effort should be made to distinguish between wall nodularity and the hyperechogenic foci within the wall. The latter when present in lesion with low level echoes and no features of malignancy is indicative of endometrioma.

Differential diagnoses of chocolate cyst include haemorrhagic cyst, dermoid cyst and cystic neoplasms. Dermoid cyst usually exhibit either echogenic shadow due to its fat content or acoustic shadowing due to calcium which aids in the diagnosis. To differentiate between haemorrhagic cyst and chocolate cyst can be a difficult task. The haemorrhagic cyst usually displays high level internal echoes within a thin walled cyst which may advance with time and emerge as a more complex cyst. Formation of fibrin may imitate thin septa but these lesions usually resolve on follow up.

The accuracy of USG can be further improved by color Doppler flow studies. Blood flow in the endometrioma is through the regularly spaced vessels running in the hilar region and the pericystic space.

MRimaging is another tool for identifying endometriomas. Due to the cyclical bleeding endometriomas contain blood products at different age. They are seen as bright or hyperintense lesions on T1 weighted image. On T2 they appear more hypointense or dark with foci of hyperintensity, imparting it the classical appearance of 'shading'. Shading is effect of degenerated blood products present at different stage within the same cyst. It can range from subtle layering to a complete signal void (black).

Since both the haemorrhagic cysts and the chocolate cyst contain blood products, it can be difficult to distinguish between them except for the fact that hemorrhagic cysts do not display shading, are mostly unilocular and resolve on interval imaging. In contrast dermoid cysts are easily diagnosed on MRI since they lose the signals and become dark on fat suppressed sequences.

After contrast administration, the periovarian peritoneal surface of the cyst can be enhanced which can help in identification of torsion ovary. Endometrioma in an enlarged but poorly enhancing ovary with peripherally located follicles is suggestive of torsion ovary on MRimaging.

5.3 Solid deep lesions

Solid deep lesions display low to intermediate signal intensity with punctuate areas of high signal intensity on T1 weighted images. Uniform low signal intensity is seen on T2 weighted images. The punctuate foci of high intensity are due to the zone of haemorrhage surrounded by abundant solid fibrous tissues. These may actually mimic metastatic lesions arising from intraperitoneal malignancies such as ovarian carcinomas. The two entities can be differentiated on T2 weighted images by the low signal intensity imparted by solid endometriomas often in combination with the presence of endometrial cyst.

Masses situated in the pouch of Douglas, posterior vaginal fornix and uterosacral ligaments may comprise of large fraction of glandular material with little fibrotic reaction, imparting hyperintense signals on T2 weighted images. Administration of contrast material will enhance such solid lesions, making it possible to distinguish it from necrosis or intramural hemorrhage.

Frequently the signal intensity may not be able to pick up the deep endometriosis of the uterosacral ligaments, especially if the punctuate foci of haemorrhage are missing in the lesion. In such case, the diagnosis is often made by correlating the thickening of the ligaments. Thickening more than 9mm in size or nodularity within the ligaments either bilateral or asymmetrical often give clue to the diagnosis.

5.4 Bladder endometriosis

Bladder endometriosis can be identified on MRI by deviation in signal intensity and gross anatomical anomalies in bladder wall thickness which can be localized or diffuse. Most of the times there are foci of high signal intensity in abnormally thickened bladder wall. Such findings may exist even if patients have normal cystoscopy result or without urinary symptoms. Bladder endometriosis infact infrequently infilterates the mucosa. Thus it is difficult to make out the lesions on cystoscopy. Advanced disease may present as ureteral obstruction and hydronephrosis.

5.5 Rectal endometriosis

Deep rectal involvement is less obvious on MRimaging due to the rectal contents which impart artifacts. Conventional MRI has infact sensitivity of only 33%. Results can be

improved with the use of phased array coils, endovaginal coils and rectal contrast enema.
MRI features that can be helpful in diagnosis include thickening of the rectal wall correlated
with specific symptoms clinically, low signal intensity on T2 weighted images, and
occasionally the presence of punctuate hyperintense foci of haemorrhage.

Endorectal sonography as dicussed earlier is superior to MR imaging for diagnosis of this
entity. The deposits on bowel are seen as rounded hypoechoic areas.

5.6 Malignant transformation in endometriosis

Malignant transformation in endometrioma is a rare well-known complication of
endometriosis, occurring in a younger age group with estimated incidence is less than 1% of
women with ovarian endometriosis. The common histologic types are endometrioid
adenocarcinoma and clear cell carcinoma arising from glandular elements and rare form is
endometrial stromal sarcoma occurs arising from stromal elements. Loss of the T2 shading
effect is more commonly detected in malignant than in benign endometriomas. The
postulated reasoning for this is dilution of haemorrhagic fluid by tumor secretions, although
is not specific to malignant endometrial cysts. Enhancing mural nodules within a cystic
mass is another feature of malignant change in endometriosis. Typically mural nodules are
enhancing, T1-weighted low and variable T2-weighted signal intensities. Dynamic
subtraction images with a gradient- echo sequence often improve nodule enhancement.
Again, enhancing mural nodules within endometriotic cysts, although seen more commonly
in malignant endometriomas is not specific and has been reported in benign lesions.

5.7 Scar endometriosis

Solid endometriosis can also develop in a caesarian section scar. MRI is valuable in
identifying these lesions. MRI characteristically shows high signal intensity on T1 and
hypointensity on T2 weighted images. Fat saturated sequences are more helpful in the
diagnosis specially in context of myometrium along the surgical scar.

6. Conclusion

The imaging techniques have revolutionized the pre operative diagnosis of endometriosis
although the ultimate confirmation is by histopathology only. The major advantage of these
tools is being non invasive method.

7. References

Gougoutas CA, Siegelman ES, Hunt J, et al. Pelvic endometriosis: various manifestations
and MR imaging findings. AJR Am J Roentgenol2000; 175: 353-358.

Knonickx PR, Meulman C, Demeyere S, Lesaffre E, CornillieFJ. Suggestive evidence that
pelvic endometriosis is a progressive disease, whereas deeply infiltrating
endometriosis is associated with pelvic pain. Fertil Steril 1991; 55: 759-765.

Patel MD, Feldstein VA, Chen DC, Lipson SD et al. Endometriomas: diagnostic performance
of US. Radiology 1999; 210: 739-745.

Stratton P, Winkel C, Premkumar A et al. Diagnostic accuracy of laparoscopy, magnetic resonance imaging, and histopathologic examimation for the detection of endometriosis. Fertil Steril 2003; 79: 1078-1085

11

Medical Treatment in Endometriosis

Elham Pourmatroud
Ahvaz Jundishapur University of Medical Science (AJUMS),
Iran

1. Introduction

Two important targets from medical treatment are: pain control and suppression of disease progress. Most of the time, the effectiveness is temporary and lasted while these drugs have been used, which is expected from the nature of endometriosis disease .Of course, there are some debts about the usefulness of pain relief agents, because 30-50% of patients feel better with placebo administration.

It must to keep in mind that those common administrated drugs couldn't help to restore the fertility potentials and in fact during their usage pregnancy cannot or should not be happened, regarding to inhibition of ovulation or teratogenic effects; of course by their administration with remission of disease (suppress the growth and activity of previous endometriotic implants) and reducing the chance of new peritoneal seeding, fertility may be preserved better; but at the end for achieving pregnancy other ways should be used.

Medical therapeutic drugs divided in two categories:

a. Non hormonal medical therapy.
b. Hormonal medical therapy.

Non hormonal therapeutic options, mainly work on inflammatory and immunologic aspect of endometriosis and hormonal attempts basically deprived endometriotic implants from their nutritive substance: estrogen.

2. Non hormonal medical therapy

2.1 Non-steroidal anti- inflammatory agents

With attention to inflammatory nature of endometriosis, for decades non- steroidal anti-inflammatory agents (NSAIDs) such as naproxen and ibuprofen have been administrated for pain control, in endometriosis. These drugs have been reduced prostaglandins (PGs) production, the main stimulator factor in peritoneal nerves and decrease the nociceptor input messenger from the peritoneal endometriotic implants into central nervous system. Their gastrointestinal upsets and inhibition of ovulation (Duffy &Stouffer,2002) against low cost and easy availability, always puts NSAIDs in a challenging situation; rather than, new NSAIDs as a selective cyclooxygenase (COX)-2 inhibitors like celecoxib without any effect on PG pathway, could induce apoptosis in endometriotic implants (Seo etal,2010). However the latest Cochrane review doesn't show significant effective role of these drugs in patients with endometriosis (Davis etal, 2007).

2.2 Cytokines inhibitors

Research in this field is still in primary stages. In animal experiments, cytokines antagonist agents like recombinant human tumor necrotizing factor alpha (TNF-α) binding protein could inhibit the progress of endometriotic implants and formation of their adhesion (Barrier etal,2004;D'Hooghe etal,2006). Etanercept (ETA) as a TNF antagonist could decrease the volume of peritoneal fluid and proliferation of lesions in endometriotic rats (Zulfikaroglu etal,2011). In a novel study, has been found that TNF could activate estrogen receptor α (ERα); therefore co-administration of a pure ER antagonist with TNF inhibitor could be a more efficacious therapeutic method than usage of one agent, separately (Gori etal,2011).

2.3 New anti inflammatores

In cases with persistent non responsive symptom to NSAIDs, other inflammatores like leukotrienes could be inhibited (Abu etal, 2000). In one new study, leukotriene receptor antagonist has been shown to have a significant effect in reduction of stromal proliferation in endometriotic implants (Ihara etal, 2004).

2.4 Immuno modulators

Pentoxiphylline administration in human, like a leukotriene receptor antagonist, had promising results in patients with endometriosis. Although it is famous as a vasodilator agent and increase tissue oxygenation in some disease; but could change the immune cell function by inhibition of cytokine and TNF-α secretion. Although in a Cochran review in year 2009, there were not shown enough evidence to support any differences in pregnancy rate in treated patients in comparison with placebo (Lu etal,2009); but in a new report, Vascular endothelial growth factor (VEGF)-C suggested to be an effective factor for significant reduction in endometriotic implants after Pentoxiphylline administration (Vlahos etal,2010).

Also, other immuno modulators like etanercept (ETA) had promising reductive effect equally to letrozole in early investigation (Ceyhan etal ,2011).

2.5 Alternative medicine

In a 16 weeks prospective clinical trial, Chinese herbal medicine (CHM) decoctions have been disclosed hopeful reduction in patient's symptoms especially with dysmenorrhea complaint rather than placebo (Flower etal, 2011). According to Cochrane review, CHM have been shown equal results in comparison with gestrinone with lesser side effects; beside that, the combination of oral CMH administration with a CMH enema appear better clinical outcomes (Flower etal, 2009).

As well, there are some published studies about the effectiveness of acupuncture in abdominal pain and significantly in dysmenorrhea relief (M.Chen etal ,2010 ; Rubi-Klein etal,2010). In another clinical trial, abdominal acupuncture causing decrease in CA125 level in endometriotic patients (Xiang etal, 2011).

3. Hormonal medical therapy

3.1 Oral contraceptive pill (OCP)

Oral combined contraceptive pills induce atrophy in peritoneal endometriotic implants by initial decidualization effect like a pseudo pregnancy situation; perhaps they could increase the apoptosis in endometriotic implants (Meresman etal , 2000). OCPs are the most prescripted drugs in endometriosis, especially in minimal and mild stages of disease for pain control ; although there is a new report about the effectiveness of OCPs usage in patients with deep endometriotic nodules (advance stage) (Mabrouk etal,2011) ,which eliminate the effectiveness of OCPs administration only in early stages of disease. In addition, there is not any differences between various available formulations in pain relief potency and any kind of OCPs which had 30-35µg of ethinyl estradiol could be used and there is no necessity for high dose (HD) contraceptive administration (with 50 µg of ethinyl estradiol) (Davis etal,2007) . About the usage methods has been shown that, continues usage had better clinical results rather than cyclic administration (Harada etal,2008). In cases of sever atrophy of endometrium and break through bleeding, supplemental estrogen for 7-10 days could be advised.

3.2 Progestins

Progestins at the first stage of administration induce decidualization in endometriotic tissues and at the second phase by proliferation inhibition makes atrophia. Also, progestins make depletion in estrogen receptors and inhibit their activation (Kirkland etal, 1992). Progestins could induce transformation of potent form of estrogens (estradiol) to weaker product (estrone) (Tseng etal, 1981) .In recent studies discover that there are two important catalyzer enzymes which metabolize progesterone in endometriotic implants. Aldo-Keto reductase 1C1 and 1C3 (AKR1C1 & AKR1C3) had significant up-regulation expression in ovarian endometriosis which interfere with inhibitory effects of human progesterone (Hevir etal, 2011). It found that exogenous progestins administration could inhibit their activity (Beranic etal, 2011).Various available progestins could be used: oral, parenteral, intrauterine device and implants. With higher dosage of administrated progestins, another effective role of them could be achieved: inhibition of matrix metalloproteinase (Osteen etal , 2003). Most of the time the clinical response to progestins are like the oral contraceptive pills (Schlaff etal,2006), without significant side effects except breakthrough bleeding which can be managed with short time, low dose estrogen administration. Also, the probably bone loss effect is reversible (Cundy etal,1996).The levonorgestrel releasing intrauterine device (LNG-IUS) is a valuable therapeutic option especially for women with deep infiltrative endometriotic implants (Lochat etal,2005).About the pain relief efficacy of progestin subdermal implants (Implanon) evidences are limited than other therapeutic modalities (Yisa etal,2005).

3.3 Gonadotropin-releasing hormone agonists

Gonadotropin –releasing hormone (GnRH) agonists are synthetic drugs which are resistant to degeneration in body and are produced by some variation in amino acids consequent in natural GnRH agonists. Their resistance to degeneration makes the pituitary gland into down regulation state and after suppression of FSH and LH production, menstruation and ovulation had been stopped and therefore, low estrogenic environment achieved which inhibits the proliferation in endometriotic implants. Beside initial flare effect, pseudo menopausal situation produce minor side effects like hot flashes, vaginal atrophia and dryness, headache and other vasomotor signs and symptoms (Dlugi etal,1990) which could be managed by add-back therapy, but after 6 or more continues cycles of drug administration, bone mineral density is going to be reduced sometimes in an irreversible manner (Taga etal,1996); but there is an interesting report about ten years usage of GnRH agonist with add-back therapy without any bone mineral loss (Bedaiwy etal,2006). Unlike the progestins and danazole, GnRH agonists had not adverse effects on lipid profile (Burry etal,1989).Several kinds of injectable GnRH agonists and nasal spray form are available with equal efficacy (Prentice etal,2000).

3.4 Gonadotropin-releasing hormone antagonists

Regarding to initial flare effect of GnRH agonist administration and probably exacerbation effect on endometriosis and a delay between their administration and real hypo estrogenic state and their intolerable side effects in some patients, GnRH antagonists became an suitable substitute for GnRH agonists. Weekly subcutaneous 3-mg cetrotide (GnRH antagonist) injection had been shown clinical efficacy without pseudo menopausal side effects (Finas etal, 2006; Kupker etal, 2002).There are some published advances in oral GnRH antagonist production: Elagolix (C.Chen et al, 2008). In a double blind study in 55 patients, weekly usage of this drug , results effective suppression of gonadal hormonal production (Struthers etal,2009), which could be a promising development in endometriosis treatments modalities instated of injectable options.

3.5 Androgens

Danazol is a derivation from testosterone which effect on endometriosis from several ways. Danazol inhibit some steroidogenic enzymes and elevate free testosterone and reduce estrogen level (Barbieri etal, 1981). Also, danazol inhibit mid cycle LH surge (Tamura etal, 1991) and PG F2α production in ovary (Kogo etal,1992),which both of them result chronic anovulation and decrease the chance of new peritoneal seeding.Danazol with 400-800 mg/daily recommended dosage regress the endometriotic implants (Telimaa etal,1987), but severe side effects prevent such dosage administration for an effective period (6 months) (Miller etal,1998).Oily skin, acne, hirsutism, irreversible voice deepness, variation in lipid profile, vaginal atrophia and hot flash limited it's prescription (Hayashi etal,2001).

3.6 Aromatase inhibitors

In opposition to other hormonal therapeutic options which reduce ovarian estrogenic production, aromatase inhibitors act not only locally on endometriotic implants, but also on all of estrogenic producers: ovary, brain, adipose tissues (Attar&Bulun, 2006). Anastrazole 1mg or letrozole 2.5mg daily could be effective in pain relief associated with endometriosis (Nothnick, 2011; Shippen&West, 2004). Because of stimulatory action of aromatase inhibitors in FSH secretion, in premenopausal women they could cause ovarian cysts;

therefore they administrate with GnRH agonist or OCPs or progestins. This method could reduce the concern about their disadvantage in prolong usage: bone loss (Ferrero etal ,2009).

3.7 Prolactin secretion inhibitors

Suppression of cellular immunity and NK cell activity in endometriotic patients has been well known. Also, in stressful situations inhibition of NK cell had been found (Chrousos etal, 2000). Prolactin and cortisol levels in serum are stress indicators. Of course the mechanism of hyper prolactinemia in response to stress isn't so clear, elevated level of serum prolactin had been found in endometriosis like other stressful conditions (Lima etal, 2006, Wang etal, 2009). Interestingly the mean serum prolactin levels are higher in advance stages in endometriotic patients (Gregoriou etal ,1999). Quinagolide as a dopamine receptor 2 agonist by reduction in VEGF receptor (a main factor for angiogenesis) could decrease the size of peritoneal lesions and in some cases could eradicate all of endometriotic implants (Gomez etal, 2011). From another aspect quinagolide, is a valuable option for hyper prolactinemia like other dopamine agonists (bromocriptine or caberguline) (Barlier&Jaquet,2006); therefore this drug could be effectively administrated in endometriosis.

4. References

Abu JI, Konje JC (2000). Leukotrienes in gynecology: the hypothetical value of anti-leukotriene therapy in dysmenorrhea and endometriosis. Hum Reprod Update, Vol. 6, PP.200-205

Attar E, Bulun S (2006). Aromatase inhibitors: the next generation of therapeutics for endometriosis? Fertil Steril, Vol. 85, PP.1307-18

Barbieri RL, Osathanondh R& Ryan KJ (1981). Danazol inhibition of steroidogenesis in the human corpus luteum .ObstetGynecol,Vol. 57, P. 722

Barlier A, Jaquet P (2006). Quinagolide a valuable treatment option for hyper prolactinemia. Eur J Endocrinol,Vol.154, No.2, PP.187-95

Barrier BF, Bates WB, Leland MM, et al (2004).Efficacy of anti-tumor necrosis factor therapy in the treatment of spontaneous endometriosis in baboons.FertilSteril, Vol.81, PP.775-79

Bedaiwy MA, Casper RF (2006).Treatment with leuprolide acetate and hormonal add-back for up to 10 years in stage 4 endometriosis patients with chronic pelvic pain.FertilSteril, Vol.86, PP.220-222

BeranicN,Gobec S&Rizner TL (2011).Progestins as inhibitors of the human 20-Ketosteroid reductase, AKR1C1 and AKR1C3.ChemBiol Interact, Vol.191,No.1-3,PP.227-33

Burry KA, Patton PE& Illingworth DR (1989). Metabolic changes during medical treatment of endometriosis: nafarelin acetate versus danazol, Am J ObstetGynecol , Vol.160, P.1454

Ceyhan ST, Onguru O, Fidan U, et al (2011).Comparison of aromatase inhibitor (letrozole) and immuno modulators (infliximab and etanercept) on regression of endometriotic implants in a rat model.Eur J ObstetGynecolReprodBiol , Vol.154, No.1, PP.100-4

Chen C, WU D, Guo Z, et al (2008). Discovery of R-(+)-4-{2-[5-(2- fluoro-3-methyl-2,6-dioxo-3,6-dihdro-2H-pyrimidin-1-yI]-1- phenylethylamino} butyrate (elgolix), a potent and orally available nonpeptide antagonist of the human gonadotropin releasing hormone receptor. J Med Chem, Vol.51,No.23, PP.7478-85

Chen M, Zhang H, Li J, et al (2010). Clinical observation on acupuncture combined with acupoint sticking therapy for treatment of dysmenorrhea caused by endometriosis. Zhongguo Zhen Jiu,Vol.30,No.9,PP.725-8

Chrousos GP, Elenkov IJ (2000).Interactions of the endocrine and immune systems. In: DeGroot LJ, Jameson JL (Editors), Endocrinology. New York: Academic Press ,PP. 571-586

Cundy T, Farquhar CM, Cornish J, etal (1996). Short-term effects of high dose oral medroxyprogesterone acetate on bone density in premenopausal women. J ClinEndocrinolMetab, Vol.81,P.1014

Davis L, Kennedy SS, Moore J, etal (2007). Modern combined oral contraceptives for pain associated with endometriosis. Cochrane Database Syst Rev.CD001019

D'Hooghe TM, Nugent N, Cuneo S, et al (2006). Recombinant human TNF binding protein (r-hTBP-1) inhibits the development of endometriosis in baboons: a prospective, randomized, placebo- and drug-controlled study. Biology of Reproduction. Vol.74, PP.131-36

Dlugi AM, Miller JD&Knittle J (1990). Lupron depot (leuprolide acetate for depot suspension) in the treatment of endometriosis: a randomized, placebo-controlled, double-blind study. Lupron Study Group, Fertil Steril .Vol.54,P.419

Duffy DM, Stouffer R .(2002). Follicular administration of a cyclooxygenase inhibitor can prevent oocyte release without alteration of normal luteal function in rhesus monkeys. HUM Reprod.V0l.17, PP.2825-31

Ferrero S, Camerini G, Seracchioli R, et al (2009). Letrozole combined with norethisterone acetate compared With norethisterone acetate alone in the treatment of pain symptoms caused by endometriosis. Hum Reprod.Vol.24,PP.3033

Flower A, Liu JP, Chen S, etal (2009).Chinese herbal medicine for endometriosis. Cochrane Database Syst Rev .Vol.8, No.3,CD006568

Flower A, Lewith GT& Little P (2011).A feasibility study exploring the role of Chinese herbal medicine in the treatment of endometriosis. J Altern Complement Med. Vol.17, No.8,PP.691-9

Finas D, Hornung D, DiedrichK,etal (2006).Cetrolix in the treatment of female infertility and endometriosis. Expert OpinPhamacother . Vol.7, No.15, PP.2155-68

Gomez R, Abad A, Delgado F, et al (2011). Quinagolide on endometriotic lesions in patients with endometriosis associated hyper prolactinemia. FertilSteril, Vol.95,N0.3,PP.882-88

Gori I, Pellegrini C, Staedler D, et al (2011). Tumor necrosis factor-α activates estrogen signaling pathways in endometrial epithelial cells via estrogen receptor α. Mol Cell Endocrinol,Vol.345,No.1-2,PP:27-37

Gregoriou G, Bakas P, Vitoratos N, et al (1999). Evaluation of serum prolactin levels in patients with endometriosis and infertility. Gynecol Obstet Invest , Vol.48, PP.48-51

Harada T, Momoeda M, Taketani Y, etal (2008). Low-dose oral contraceptive pill for dysmenorrhea associated with endometriosis: a placebo-controlled, double-blind, randomized trial,FertilSteril.Vol.90,P.1583

Hayashi T, Takahashi T, Minami T, et al (2001). Fatal acute hepatic failure induced by danazol in a patient with endometriosis and aplastic anemia. J Gastroenterol. Vol.36,PP. 783-86

Hevir N, Vouk K, Sinkovec J, etal (2011). Aldo-KetoReductases AKR1C1, AkR1C2 and AKR1C3 may enhance progesterone metabolism in ovarian endometriosis. ChemBiol Interact .Vol.191,No.1-3,PP.217-26

Ihara T, Uchiide I&Sugamata M (2004).Light and electron microscopic evaluation of antileukotriene therapy for experimental rat endometriosis.FertilSteril .Vol.81, suppl.1,PP.819-23

Kirkland JL, Murthy L&Stancel GM (1992).Progesterone inhibits the estrogen-induced expression ofc-fos messenger ribonucleic acid inthe uterus, Endocrinology .Vol.130,P.3223

Kogo H, Takasaki K, Yatabe Y, etal (1992). Inhibitory and stimulatory actions of danazol in rat ovarian and uterine tissues. Eur J Pharmacol, Vol.211, No.1,PP.69-73

Kupker W, Felberbaum RE, Krapp M, etal (2002).Use of GnRH antagonists in the treatment of endometriosis.Reprod Biomed Online, Vol.5,No.1, PP.12-16

Lima A.P, Rosa e Silva A.A.M (2006).Prolactin and cortisol levels in women with endometriosis. Brazilian J of Med BiolRes ,Vol.39, PP.1121-27

Lochat FB, Emembolu JO&Konje JC (2005).The efficacy, side effects and continuation rates in women with symptomatic endometriosis undergoing treatment with an intrauterine administered progesterone (levonorgestrone) :a 3 –year follow –up. Hum Reprod, Vol.20, PP.789-793

LU D, Song H, Li Y, etal (2009).Pentoxiphylline versus medical therapies for sub fertile women with endometriosis. Cochrane Database Of Systemic Reviews .Issue 3.Art. No:CD007677

Mabrouk M, Frasca C, Geraci E, et al (2011).Combined oral contraceptive therapy in women with posterior deep infiltrating endometriosis. J Minim Invasive Gynecol, Vol.18, No.4,PP.470-4

Meresman GF, Vighi S, Buquet RA, etal (2000). Apoptosis and expression of Bcl-2 and Bax in eutopic endometrium from women with endometriosis. FertilSteril. Vol.74,P.760

Miller JD, Shaw RW, Casper RF, et al (1998). Historical prospective cohort study of the recurrence of pain after discontinuation of treatment with danazol or a gonadotropin-releasing hormone agonist.FertilSteril. Vol.70,P.293

Nothnick WB (2011).The emerging use of aromatase inhibitors for endometriosis treatment.ReprodBiolEnocrinol,Vol.9,P.87

Osteen KG, Igarashi TM& Bruner-Tran KL (2003). Progesterone action in the human endometrium: induction of a unique tissue environment which limits matrix metalloproteinase (MMP) expression, Front Biosci,Vol.8,P.d78

Prentice A, Deary AJ, Goldbeck-Wood S, etal (2000). Gonadotropin- releasing hormone analogues for pain associated with endometriosis, Cochrane Database Syst Rev .CD000346

Rubi-Klein K, Kucera-Sliutz E, Nissel H, et al (2010). Is acupuncture in addition to conventional medicine effective as pain treatment for endometriosis? A randomized controlled cross-over trial.Eur J ObstetGynecolReprodBiol,Vol.153, No.1,PP.90-3

Schlaff WD, Carson SA, Luciano A, et al (2006). Subcutaneous injection of depot medroxyprogesterone acetate compared with leuprolide acetate in the treatment of endometriosis –associated pain. Hum Reprod,Vol. 21,PP.248-256

SeoSk, Nam A, Jeon YE, et al (2010).Expression and possible role of non-steroidal anti-inflammatory drug-activated gene-1 (NAG-1) in the human endometrium and endometriosis. Hum Reprod,Vol.25, N0.12, PP. 3043-9

Shippen ER, West WJ, Jr (2004).Successful treatment of severe endometriosis in two premenopausal women with an aromatase inhibitor.FertilSteril, Vol.81,P.1395

Struthers RS, Nicholls AJ, Grundy J, et al (2009).Suppression of gonadotropins and estradiol in premenopausal women by oral administration of the nonpeptide gonadotropin releasing hormone antagonist elagolix. J ClinEndocrinolMetab, Vol.94, No.2,PP.545-51

Taga M, Minaguchi H (1996). Reduction of bone mineral density by gonadotropin-releasing hormone agonist, nafarelin, is not completely reversible at 6 months after the cessation of administration. Acta Obstet Gynecol Scand,Vol.75,P.162

Tamura K, Okamoto R, Takeo S, etal (1991).Inhibition of the first ovulation and ovarian prostaglandin F2 alpha metabolism by danazol in rats.Eur JPharmacol, Vol.202,No.3,PP.317-22

Telimaa S, Puolakka J, RonnbergL,etal (1987). Placebo controlled Comparison of danazol and high-dose medroxyprogesterone acetate in the treatment of endometriosis, GynecolEndocrinol , Vol.1, P.13

Tseng L, Lui HC (1981). Stimulation of arylsulfotransferase activity by progestins in human endometrium in vitro, J ClinEndocrinolMetab, Vol.53,P.418

Vlahos NF, Grogoriou O, Deliveliotou A, et al (2010).Effect of Pentoxiphylline on vascular endothelial growth factor c and flk-1 expression on endometrial implants in the rat endometriosis model.FertilSteril,vol.93,No.4,PP.1316-23

Wang H, GorpudoloN&Behr B   (2009).The role of prolactin and endometriosis associated infertility. ObstetGynecolSurv,Vol.64, No.8,PP.542-7

Xiang DF, Sun QZ &Liang XF (2011). Effect of abdominal acupuncture on pain of pelvic cavity in patients with endometriosis . Zhongguo Zhen Jiu,Vol.31,No.2, PP.113-6

Yisa SB, Okenwa AA &Husemeyer RP (2005).Treatment of pelvic endometriosis with etonogestrel subdermal implant (Implanon). J FamPlannReprod Health Care ,vol.31,PP.67-70

Zulfikaroglu E, Kilic S, Islimye M, et al (2011).Efficacy of anti-tumor necrosis factor therapy on endometriosis in an experimental rat model.RchGynecolObstet,Vol.283, No.4, PP.799-804

12

Pathophysiological Changes in Early Endometriosis

Tao Zhang, Gene Chi Wai Man and Chi Chiu Wang
Department of Obstetrics and Gynaecology, The Chinese University of Hong Kong,
Prince of Wales Hospital, Shatin, New Territories,
Hong Kong

1. Introduction

Endometriosis is a common but complex gynecological disorder of unknown pathogenesis. It is characterized by ectopic growth of endometrial tissues. Based on Sampson's classical implantation theory, retrograde menstruation, immune escape, adhesion, angiogenesis and growth of endometrial cells are essential milestones in the pathogenesis of endometriosis. The cellular communications of immune, endothelial and endometriotic cells during endometriosis development are mediated via cytokines and chemokines. Many specific cytokines in peritoneal fluid of patients with endometriosis are aberrant from normal women. However, it's not clear at which stage of endometriosis these aberrant cytokines begin to change and owing to the limitation with human study the functions of these cytokines were only investigated in vitro. On the other hand, the onset of angiogenesis is initiated by oxidative stress due to cellular and tissue hypoxia, which is mainly coordinated by the hypoxia-inducible factors (HIFs). HIFs stimulate VEGF transcription and activation in endometriosis lesions in acquiring new blood vessels for survival and growth. Monitoring inflammatory response, oxidative stress and angiogenesis in the endometriosis lesions is of vital importance in understanding the pathophysiological changes during early development of endometriosis.

In our studies, we investigated for the first time the dynamic changes of oxygen reactive species and angiogenesis in the endometriosis implants by in vivo imaging techniques and characterized regulation of cytokines, hypoxia and angiogenesis factors within the first 24 hour of experimental endometriosis in mice. We identified significant oxidative stress and hypoxia responses in the endometriosis implants in early phase only, but specific estrogen-dependent cytokine activations and angiogenesis signaling in late phase. In this chapter, we will describe the non-invasive in vivo imaging method as a valuable tool for monitoring oxidative stress and angiogenesis in endometriosis and to understand its role in the early development and growth of endometriosis. We will also demonstrate oxidative stress preceded hypoxia and cytokine activation and angiogenesis signaling in the pathogenesis of early endometriosis.

2. Development of endometriosis

2.1 Sampson's implantation theory

Endometriosis is one of most common gynecological disorder, but poorly understood condition. As early as in 1860, von Rokitansky (Rokitansky, 1860) is the first one to describe this disease in detail. Since then, several postulated theories explaining the pathogenesis of endometriosis were raised. The most popular theory is Sampson's classical implantation theory in 1921 (Sampson, 1921). He proposed that the endometrial fragments of uterine endometrium during menstruation can regurgitate through the fallopian tubes and survive in the peritoneal cavity, developing to endometriosis.

There have been numerous studies in human and primate support the implantation theory (Bartosik et al., 1986; Halme et al., 1984). However, this hypothesis cannot explain why only about 10% women suffer from endometriosis, but the incidence of retrograde menstruation should be much higher. What's more, the endometriotic lesion sometimes is present out of peritoneal cavity, such as lungs, brain and heart, instead of peritoneal cavity only (Felson et al., 1960; Joseph et al., 1994; Thibodeau et al., 1987). Besides, genetic, immunological factors and vascular and lymphatic spread are also essential for endometriosis development. Therefore, endometriosis is multifactorial and complicated condition. More studies are needed to explicitly understand the pathogenesis of endometriosis.

2.2 Pathophysiology

With numerous clinical and basic researches on endometriosis, especially peritoneal endometriosis, based on Sampson's retrograde menstruation theory, it's well accepted that the appearance of vital endometrial cells is the first step. Then immune escape, adhesion, implantation, angiogenesis and proliferation are all very important during the development of endometriosis (Fig. 1).

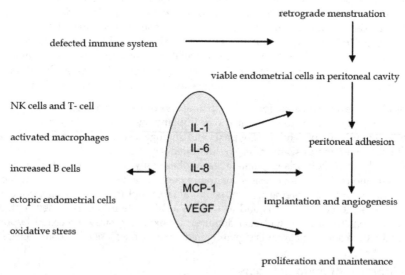

Fig. 1. Summary of the development of endometriosis

In healthy women, macrophages, lymphocytes, natural killer cells and leukocytes eliminate ectopic endometrial cells (Braun *et al.*, 1996). Though the number of immune cells in peritoneal fluid of women with endometriosis was significantly higher than women without this disease, the function of increased immune cells was decreased (Berkkanoglu *et al.*, 2003). Meanwhile, these defected immune cells may secrete some cytokines and growth factors, such as interleukin-1 (IL-1), interleukin-8 (IL-8), monocyte chemotactic protein 1 (MCP-1) and vascular endothelial growth factor (VEGF) etc., which may help the endometrial cells escape from immune surveillance to adhere to the peritoneum, establish microvessels and finally grow under the stimulation of estrogen cycle (Kyama *et al.*, 2003). However, the reasons causing impaired immune cells are not known. When and what kind of cells as well as molecules taking part in the process from survival to steady growth are still not clear.

2.3 Cellular communications

Endometrial cells have to contact with immune cells, peritoneal lining and vascular endothelial before final growth and maintenance in ectopic location. Cellular immune response is responsible for implantation of the retrograde and vital endometrial cells. The molecules secreted by immune cells would effect the reaction between endometrial cells and other cells.

2.3.1 Macrophages

Macrophages are the most abundant immune cells in peritoneal fluid and their main role is to phagocytose cellular debris and pathogens. They can also promote lymphocytes and other immune cells to respond to pathogens (Tariverdian *et al.*, 2009; van Furth *et al.*, 1979). It has been reported that the number and activity of macrophages in peritoneal fluid significantly increased. However they cannot clear the ectopic endometrial cells and inhibit the development of endometriosis. Modulators of activated macrophages for both immune and non-immune cells promote growth and maintenance of ectopic lesion (Lebovic *et al.*, 2001). There are several evidence to support the change of receptors expression on macrophages leads to impaired scavenger function, which might be caused by abnormal cytokines and growth factors in the peritoneal fluid of women with endometriosis (Berkkanoglu *et al.*, 2003).

2.3.2 Lymphocytes

The two main types of lymphocytes are: B cells accounting for humoral acquired response by secreting soluble antibodies into the body's fluids for eliminating foreign antigens, and T cells responsible for cellular responses. Both of which recognize specific antigen targets. T cells are mainly differentiated into helper T cells promoting antibody production secreted by B cells, regulatory T cells controlling immune response, and cytotoxic/suppressor T cells killing infected cells and cancer cells in the thymus. In endometriosis, it was reported that the proliferation and cytotoxic activity of lymphocytes in peripheral blood is decreased (Dmowski *et al.*, 1981; Steele *et al.*, 1984). Increased T cells, both helper and suppressor T cells, in peritoneal fluid and ectopic endometriotic tissue was observed in women with endometriosis (Dmowski *et al.*, 1994; Hill *et al.*, 1988; Mettler *et al.*, 1996). However, the changes are not consistent. Besides, the function and activity of peripheral T cells might be different from those in peritoneal fluid. In all, it's controversial if the alteration of lymphocytes in peripheral and peritoneal fluid play a role in the development of endometriosis.

2.3.3 Natural killer cells

Natural killer cells (NK cells) constitute a major component of the innate immune system. They have two ways to take part in host defense by expressing different receptors binding to target cells. One receptor type binds immunoglobulin G (IgG). The other includes killer-activating receptors promoting cytotoxic activity and killer-inhibitory receptors (KIR) suppressing cytotoxic activity (Moretta et al., 1995). Oosterlynck and Wilson have found that the cytotoxic activity of peripheral and peritoneal fluid NK cells from women with endometriosis was obviously decreased with the severity of endometriosis (Oosterlynck et al., 1991; Wilson et al., 1994). The decreased NK-mediated cytotoxicity in the peritoneal fluid might contribute to the establishment of endometriosis. The mechanisms that cause aberrant NK cell cytotoxicity are unclear, but seem to be involved in KIR expression (Wu et al., 2000). In a recent study, Maeda et al. reported KIR2DL1 as the subclass of KIR overexpressed on NK cells in peripheral and peritoneal fluid of patients with endometriosis.

2.3.4 Peritoneal cells

Several adhesion moleculars were found to be expressed in endometrium, which mediate the adhesion and invasion of endometrial cells to peritoneum. Koks found that endometrium preferentially adhere to the extracellular matrix (ECM) of the peritoneum mediated by integrin (Koks et al., 2000). Endometrium expresses various integrins during menstruation shedding and the adhesion can be disrupted by blocking integrin. Integrins are cell-surface glycoproteins acting as receptors for ECM proteins. In normal eutopic endometrium, integrins are important in the interaction between glandular epithelial and stromal cells, and essential for implantation (Lessey et al., 1992). After adherence of endometrial cells to the peritoneum, local degradation of the ECM is required for invasion and implantation. Metalloproteinases (MMPs) causing ECM breakdown, tissue collapse and menstruation was up-regulated in late secretory phase (Salamonsen et al., 1996). This implies that the vital endometrial cells in peritoneal cavity during menstruation shedding already have the potential to invade into peritoneum. What's more, MMPs are present independent of the cycle phase in peritoneal and ovarian endometriosis (Salamonsen et al., 1996), which promotes endometriotic cells to infiltrate into peritoneum further although endometriosis has been established.

2.3.5 Vascular endothelial cells

The ectopic endometrial cells require an accessible blood supply to proliferate and invade through the peritoneum after escaping immune surveillance. Greater angiogenic activity have been found in the peritoneal fluid of women with endometriosis, which are modulated by growth factors and cytokines such as VEGF & IL-8 secreted by ectopic endometrial cells and defected immune cells (Oosterlynck et al., 1993). VEGF is a mitogen for endothelial cells and stimulates the proliferation of both vascular and lymphatic endothelial cells in vitro (Joukov et al., 1997) and promotes angiogenesis or hyperplasia of lymphatic vessels in vivo (Jeltsch et al., 1997). Increasing evidence indicate that VEGF plays an important role in the angiogenesis of peritoneal endometriosis (McLaren, 2000). VEGF is elevated in the peritoneal fluid and endometriotic lesion of women with endometriosis and correlated with the severity of this disease (McLaren et al., 1996). Its expression is more pronounced around red endometriotic lesions as compared with the more inactive black implants (Donnez et al., 1998).

2.4 Molecular modulations

Cellular communications in endometriosis mediated by inflammatory cytokines and growth factors is mainly regulated by nuclear factor-κB (NF-κB) signaling pathway (Fig. 2) (Gonzalez-Ramos *et al.*). NF-κB mediated gene transcription promoting inflammation, invasion, angiogenesis, and cell proliferation and inhibiting apoptosis of endometriotic cells through p50/p65 dimers and NF-κB inhibitor IκBα has been found *in vitro* and *in vivo* studies (Gonzalez-Ramos *et al.*, 2010). Constitutive activation of NF-κB has been demonstrated in endometriotic lesions and peritoneal macrophages of patients with endometriosis (Laird *et al.*, 2000). Some drugs such as GnRH blocking NF-κB have been proven efficient at reducing endometriosis-associated symptoms in women (Han *et al.*, 2003). Overload iron produced by erythrocytes from menstruation shedding and cytokines such as interleukin-1 (IL-1) and tumor necrosis factor-α (TNF-α) as well as oxidative stress stimulate NF-κB activation in macrophages and ectopic endometrial cells, which stimulates synthesis of proinflammatory cytokines, sending a positive feedback loop to the NF-κB signaling pathway. NF-κB activation enhances factors of anti-apoptosis, growth, invasion and angiogenesis as well as proinflammatory cytokines such as cyclooxygenase 2 (COX-2), vascular endothelial growth factor (VEGF), macrophage migration inhibitory factor (MIF), interleukin-1 (IL-1) and tumor necrosis factor-α (TNF-α), which promote the development of endometriosis. Intercellular adhesion molecule-1 (ICAM-1) and RANTES up-regulated by NF-κB activity could attract more macrophages to sites of inflammation.

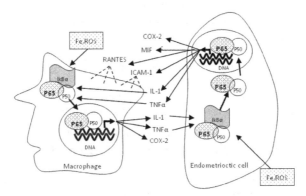

Fig. 2. NF-κB signaling pathway in endometriosis

3. Early pathogenesis

3.1 Oxidative stress

Oxidative stress has been proposed as a potential factor in the pathogenesis of endometriosis (Van Langendonckt *et al.*, 2002). Oxidative stress may occur when the balance of reactive oxygen species (ROS) and antioxidant is disturbed. Several studies have demonstrated that the oxidative stress is involved in endometriosis with increased concentration of ROS, enzymes producing ROS and lower concentration of antioxidant in peritoneal fluid and in the eutopic and ectopic endometrium of women with endometriosis (Ota *et al.*, 2001; Zeller *et al.*, 1987). It's postulated that oxidative stress is stimulated by erythrocytes (Brosens, 1994), apoptotic endometrial tissue, cell debris and macrophages (Murphy *et al.*, 1998). These inducers may cause activation and recruitment of mononuclear phagocytes which induce oxidative stress. Oxidative stress might lead to a localized pelvic inflammatory reaction with increased pro-inflammatory mediators, cytokines and growth factors (Gupta *et al.*, 2006). These cytokines and growth factors have been widely accepted to promote the immune modulation, adhesion, invasion and angiogenesis of endometriosis. Therefore, understanding of oxidative stress could give a light in the initiation and process of angiogenesis and inflammation during the development of endometriosis. However, two other studies could not find the imbalance between ROS and antioxidant in the peritoneal fluid of women with endometriosis (Ho *et al.*, 1997; Wang *et al.*, 1997). This discrepancy might be due to the use of markers of oxidative stress. Thus, further studies are needed to identify when and how oxidative stress play a role in the pathophysiology of endometriosis in particular during early development.

3.2 Proinflammatory responses

It's widely accepted that endometriosis is a pelvic inflammatory process with defected function of immune system and increased level of abnormal cytokines, chemokines and growth factors in the peritoneal fluid modulating the growth and inflammation of endometriosis. The proinflammatory cytokines and chemokines involved in development of endometriosis include IL-1, IL-6, IL-8, MCP-1 and RANTES (Table 1). These cytokines are mostly secreted by activated immune cells and endometrial cells. They act as paracrine and autocrine messengers in cellular communication. On the one hand, some of these cytokines mediate the adhesion of endometrial cells to peritoneum, such as ICAM-1 and TNF-α and promote proliferation of endometrial cells, such as IL8, as well as stimulate angiogenesis such as VEGF. On the other hand, some cytokines modulate immune cells function: transforming growth factor beta (TGF-β) inhibiting T and B lymphocytes and NK cells which may cause immune tolerance; MCP-1 activating macrophages. The imbalance and abnormal distribution of peritoneal fluid cytokines and their functions imply that inflammation plays a key role in the development of endometriosis.

Whether pelvic inflammation cause endometriosis or endometriosis results in pelvic inflammation is still not well defined. Due to the unsatisfactory diagnostic methods and the limitation of human researches, we are not able to answer this question in human because most patients have had endometriosis for an unknown disease course at the time of diagnosis. Studying endometriosis using animal models complement the understanding endometriosis in human. Chen et al. have found that the endometrial cells in the peritoneal fluid induced the production of IL-1β, TNF-α, VEGF and MCP-1 at 24 hours in the peritoneal fluid of mice. (Chen *et al.*). Similarly, IL-2, IL-4, IL-6, IL-10 and MCP-1, eosinophil chemotactic protein (eotaxin), macrophage inflammatory protein and RANTES as well as CC chemokine receptor (CCR1) were found remarkably expressed in endometriotic lesions on the 4th day in rat model by autologous transplantation of endometrial epithelial fragment to peritoneum (Umezawa *et al.*, 2008). These inflammation cytokines found in early endometriosis is consistent with those found in peritoneal fluid of women with endometriosis. Based on this finding, it can be supposed that endometrial cells in peritoneal cavity might cause inflammation mediating and promoting the development of endometriosis. More studies about early endometriosis are necessary to confirm this hypothesis.

Cytokines	Functions	References
IL-1	Activates T-lymphocytes	(Vigano et al., 1998)
	Differentiates B cells	(Lebovic et al., 2000)
	Increase IL-6, sICAM-1, IL-8 & VEGF	(Arici et al., 1993)
IL-6	Stimulate B cell activity	(Le et al., 1989)
	Differentiate T cells	(Giudice, 1994)
	Stimulate angiogenesis	(Lin et al., 2006)
IL-8	Promote proliferation of endometrial and endometriotic stromal cells	(Iwabe et al., 1998)
	Stimulate adhesion of endometrial cells to fibronectin	(Arici et al., 1998)
	Recruit neutrophils and lymphocytes	(Garcia-Velasco et al., 1999)
MCP-1	Activate macrophages	(Oral et al., 1996)
	Stimulate endometrial cell proliferation	(Arici et al., 1997)
RANTES	Attract macrophages and lymphcytes	(Khorram et al., 1993)
ICAM-1	Mediate cell adhesion	(Oral et al., 1996)
	Inhibit NK cells cytotoxicity	(Koninckx et al., 1998)
TGF-β	Attract monocytes	(Oosterlynck et al., 1994)
	Inhibit T and B lymphocytes and NK cell activity	
TNF-α	Initiate the cascade of cytokines and inflammatory response	(Laird et al., 1996)
	Increase the adherence of cultured endometrial stromal cells	(Zhang et al., 1993)
VEGF	Stimulate angiogenesis; Attract monocytes	(McLaren et al., 1996)

Table 1. Functions of cytokines and growth factors involved in endometriosis

3.3 Angiogenesis

The establishment of new blood vessels is essential in growth and survival of endometriosis. Increased angiogenic activity has been demonstrated in peritoneal fluid of women with endometriosis and strong expression of angiogenic factors has been shown in active lesions (Donnez et al., 1998; Nisolle et al., 1993). Moreover, inhibition of endometrial implants by anti-angiogenic agents or VEGF receptors (VEGFR) blocker was observed in animal studies (Dabrosin et al., 2002; Nap et al., 2004). Many anti-angiogenic compounds are studied extensively in animal models of endometriosis. Vlahos stated that pentoxifylline used in the treatment of peripheral vascular disease for many years may cause suppression of endometriotic tissue by inhibiting angiogenesis through VEGF-C and VEGFR-2 expression in rat model (Vlahos et al.). Besides, progestins already used in the treatment of endometriosis inhibit human ectopic endometrial lesions in a mouse model by regulating cysteine-rich angiogenic inducer (CYR61), basic fibroblast growth factor (bFGF) and VEGFA (Monckedieck et al., 2009). Endostain, a potent endogenous inhibitor of blood vessel growth, suppress angiogenesis by inhibiting endothelial migration without effecting normal estrous cycles (Becker et al., 2006). What's more, either selective cyclooxygenase-2 (COX-2) inhibitor or immunoconjugate molecule (Icon) suppress angiogenesis in animal models by microvessels density assessment (Krikun et al.). However, there is no study to investigate the early process of angiogenesis in endometriosis, which makes new anti-angiogenesis therapy possible for prevention of reoccurrence after surgical treatment.

4. Experimental designs

Oxidative stress, proinflammatory responses and angiogenesis of endometriosis are important during early development of endometriosis. We postulate that the refluxed endometrial tissues in peritoneal cavity could stimulate oxidative stress and proinflammatory cytokines which promote the endometriotic adhesion, angiogenesis and implantation (Fig. 3). The methods we used are complementary to each other's insufficiency (Table 2).

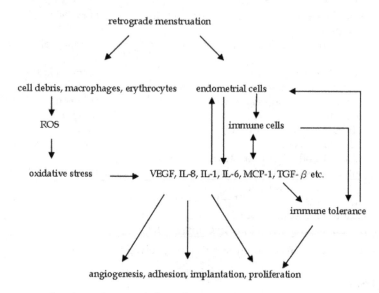

Fig. 3. Summary of early pathogenesis in endometriosis

	Method	Advantage	Disadvantage
Oxidative stress	IVIS	*in vivo*, longitudinal, semi-quantitative	Expensive
	ROS or RNS markers	*in vitro*, quantitative, sensitive	non-longitudinal, not stable
Angiogenesis	Cellvizio, IVIS	*in vivo*, longitudinal, semi-quantitative	expensive, superficial vessels
	Angiogenic markers	*in vitro*, quantitative	non-longitudinal
Cytokines	Antibody Array	small sample, all cytokines, semi-quantitative	expensive, non-longitudinal
	Multiplex	small sample, selected cytokines, quantitative	expensive, non-longitudinal
	ELISA	large sample, specific cytokines, quantitative, sensitive	non-longitudinal

Table 2. Comparison of available study methods

4.1 Oxidative stress in early endometriosis

In order to monitor the oxidative stress response in early development of endometriosis, an experimental endometriosis model in C57 mice was established by subcutaneous injection of mouse endometrium fragments. A chemiluminescent probe, L-012 (25mg/kg s.c.), was injected to the mice for the noninvasive *in vivo* oxidative stress imaging. L-012 is a new luminol derivative and sensitive chemiluminescence probe reacting with various types of ROS. ROS and reactive nitrogen species (RNS) production in the transplanted lesion can be monitored longitudinally by Xenogen IVIS 200 Imaging System. The results showed that *In vivo* imaging demonstrated significant increased bioluminescence signals for ROS/RNS from the transplanted lesions at the first hour interval. The signal reached a peak after 4 hours of transplantation. Then, the signal gradually decreased and maintained at minimal intensity in the rest of experiment. Immunohistochemistry showed positive lag correlation for the stained Hypoxia-inducible factors (HIF-1) in glandular epithelial cells and stromal tissue from the isolated lesions across the later time after transplantation. For angiogenesis, CD34, VEGF and Von Willebrand factor (vWF) signals were increased in parallel with HIF expression at 1 week thereafter. The non-invasive *in vivo* imaging method provides a valuable tool for monitoring oxidative stress in endometriosis and to understand its role in the early development and growth of endometriosis. The study indicated oxidative stress preceded HIF activation and VEGF angiogenesis in the pathogenesis of early endometriosis.

4.2 Cytokine profiling in early endometriosis

Both donor and recipient BALB/c mice at 7 weeks old were subjected to ovariectomy (OVX) and then were supplemented with 100ug/kg estradiol. Uterine horns from the donor mice were removed into F12 medium. Endometrium was punched into endometrial fragments after peeling off the serosa and myometrium under microscope. Fragments suspended in 0.3ml PBS were injected into peritoneal cavity of recipient mice. Peritoneal fluid was collected at experiment time intervals after transplantation. Cytokines profiles in peritoneal fluid were detected simultaneously. Differentially expressed cytokines were confirmed by ELISA quantification.

The results showed that the levels of CD30, CD36/SR-B3, Dickkopf-related protein (Dkk-1), epidermal growth factor (EGF), Eotaxin, IL-1 receptor antagonist (IL-1ra), IL-6 and Vascular cell adhesion protein 1 (VCAM-1) were significantly increased with the first hour of transplantation. This is the first report to analyze the peritoneal fluid cytokines profiles in experimental endometriosis in mice. The change pattern of cytokines could provide insights in understanding the early development of endometriosis. From the results, we can see that the oxidative stress and abnormal cytokine profiles might contribute to the early development of endometriosis.

4.3 Angiogenesis in early endometriosis

Mice were randomly treated with epigallocatchin-3-gallate (EGCG) extracted from green tea, Vitamin E (antioxidant controls) or vehicle (negative controls) for *in vivo* and *in vitro* microvessel imaging at the end of intervention. Microvascular networks in the endometriotic lesions *in vivo* were imaged by Cellvizio LAB LSU-488 with ProFlex Microprobe S1500. Microvessel length and area were measured using Cellvizio LAB Vessel Detection software and averaged from 4 perpendicular regions of the lesion in replicate.

Endometriotic implants were collected for angiogenesis microarray and pathway analysis after microvessel assessments *in vivo*. Differentially expressed angiogenesis molecules CD34, VEGFA, VEGFB, VEGFC, VEGFD, VEGFR1, VEGFR2 and VEGFR3 were confirmed by quantitative PCR, Western blot and immunhistochemistry. Effects of EGCG on angiogenesis signal transduction were further characterised in human endothelial cell line. Microvessel parameters and angiogenesis VEGFC/VEGFR2 signaling pathway including Jun proto-oncogene (cJUN), interferon-gamma (IFNG), matrix metallopeptidase-9 (MMP9) and chemokine (C-X-C motif) ligand-3 (CXCL3) in endometriotic implants and endothelial cells were studied. The results showed that EGCG, but not Vitamin E, inhibited microvessels in endometriotic implants. EGCG selectively suppressed VEGFC and tyrosine kinase receptor VEGFR2 expression. EGCG down regulated VEGFC/VEGFR2 signaling through cJUN, IFNG and MMP9/CXCL3 pathways for endothelial proliferation, inflammatory response and mobility. EGCG also suppressed VEGFC expression and reduced VEGFR2 and extracellular signal-regulated kinases (ERK) activation in endothelial cells. VEGFC supplementation attenuated the inhibitory effects by EGCG.

5. Prospective and proposal

5.1 Clinical significance and potential applications

Up to date, the only way to diagnose endometriosis is laparoscopy which is minimal invasive but expensive. Non-invasive and cheap diagnostic methods are urgent to be developed. CA-125 is a widely used serum marker for the diagnosis and evaluation of recurrent endometriosis or the success of a surgical treatment. A recent meta-analysis including twenty three studies and assessing the diagnostic performance of serum CA125 has shown that it's a poor diagnostic method with 90% specificity and 28% sensitivity (Mol et al., 1998). One study has found serum IL-6 and peritoneal fluid TNF-α were able to discriminate between patients with and without endometriosis (Bedaiwy et al., 2002). They stated the sensitivity and specificity of serum IL-6 reached 80% and 87% respectively, which is significantly higher than that of CA-125. It indicates that no inflammatory cytokine make a potential biomarker for diagnosis of endometriosis. Its predictive values in early endometriosis require further investigation.

In addition, the recognition of pathogenesis is able to provide new concept to the current unsatisfactory treatments. Hormone medicine is a commonly used drug for prevention of occurrence after surgical treatment. However, lots of patients are not sensitive to these medicines or cannot endure the side effects, such as vomiting and weight gain. New therapy with less adverse effects and more effective function needs to be developed. The study of oxidative stress, inflammation and angiogenesis in the pathogenesis of early endometriosis make it possible. For example, antioxidant therapy with 1200 IU of vitamin E and 1 g of vitamin C for a period of two months lead to a decrease in the inflammation cytokines such as MCP-1, RANTES and IL-6 in peritoneal fluid (Nalini Santanam, 2003). Another drug mifepristone with antioxidant effects was also found to exert an inhibitory effect on endometrial cell growth (Guo et al.). As angiogenesis, the VEGF inhibitor and anti-VEGF antibody have been demonstrated to be effective to control and inhibit implant lesion in mice model (Hull et al., 2003). As process of endometriosis contains several steps, the ideal medicine has the potential to control the development of progression of endometrium in early pathophysiological stage (Fig. 4).

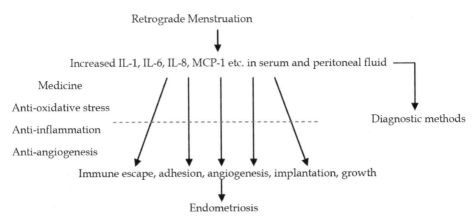

Fig. 4. Hypotheses and clinical potentials of endometriosis

5.2 Study limitations

Due to unavailable systematic studies, the understanding about this disease is still limited although endometriosis has been studied for many years. The limitations and difficulties are as below:

First, at the time of diagnosis endometriosis has already been established with unknown history. Hence, it's impossible to undertake clinical research from the onset to maintenance, which mainly makes the etiology still unknown. Second, it's difficult to have adequate control group. The control women involved in most studies are patients without endometriosis, which means they might have other disease, such as uterine myoma and benign ovarian tumor. The difference between normal eutopic and ectopic endometrium as well as normal pelvic environment and that with endometriosis is impossible to study in human. Third, we have already known genetic, immune system and peritoneal microenviroment are associated with endometriosis, which is supported by different curative effect with the same treatment for different patients and diverse symptoms. Therefore, the clinical treatment is individual and personal which increase the difficulty to observe and compare the different treatments. Fourth, only human and primates suffer from spontaneous endometriosis. The reproductive anatomy, physiology and estrogen cycle characteristics of monkeys are similar to human. Therefore, monkeys are the best animal model to do studies which can not carry out in humans. However, only few centers have the capacity to maintain this expensive animal. The most commonly used animal model is rodents, but there is an enormous phylogenetic gap between these animals and human. Hence, the question is how much data from these rodent models can be extrapolated to human situation. Fifth, primary endometrial and endometriotic epithelial cells cannot be passaged and fall into senescence within 2 weeks, but a stable cell line is necessary for the mechanism study. Until now, there are no stable and commercial normal endometrial and endometriotic glandular and stromal cells available for studying. Several researchers immortalized these cells by using human telomerase reverse transcriptase (hTERT) (Kyo et al., 2003) or transfecting SV40 T-antigen vector (Zeitvogel et al., 2001). However, how much characteristics these immortalized cells are similar to primary endometrial cells are needed to approve.

6. Conclusion

Endometriosis is a multifactorial disorder including retrograde menstruation, immune tolerance, adhesion, transplantation and proliferation modulated by abnormal inflammatory cytokines profile in peritoneal fluid. Future studies are necessary to focus on the whole picture of signaling pathway in early pathogenesis.

The current treatments mainly focus on inhibiting estrogen and its receptors which are not useful for every patient with endometriosis because estrogen is only one factor in the development of endometriosis. The signaling pathway is essential and makes it possible to develop an effective medication which could not only decrease estrogen level but also inhibit inflammation cytokines, ROS and angiogenesis. On the other hand, complete understanding of pathogenesis of endometriosis such as cytokines could provide a new way to diagnose and even to divide the disease into different stages according to pathophysiolocal characteristics, which makes the treatment individual and personal.

What's more, prevention of endometriosis after surgery is also very important. The current medicines used for prevention of recurrence are not very effective and have various side effects. The understanding of pathogenesis of early endometriosis may produce a better therapy to prevent recurrence. Ultimately, more clinical and basic researches should be carried out to overcome the complicated disease.

7. References

Arici, A, Head, JR, MacDonald, PC & Casey, ML (1993). Regulation of interleukin-8 gene expression in human endometrial cells in culture, *Mol Cell Endocrinol* 94(2): 195-204.

Arici, A, Oral, E, Attar, E, Tazuke, SI & Olive, DL (1997). Monocyte chemotactic protein-1 concentration in peritoneal fluid of women with endometriosis and its modulation of expression in mesothelial cells, *Fertil Steril* 67(6): 1065-72.

Arici, A, Seli, E, Zeyneloglu, HB, Senturk, LM, Oral, E & Olive, DL (1998). Interleukin-8 induces proliferation of endometrial stromal cells: a potential autocrine growth factor, *J Clin Endocrinol Metab* 83(4): 1201-5.

Bartosik, D, Jacobs, SL & Kelly, LJ (1986). Endometrial tissue in peritoneal fluid, *Fertil Steril* 46(5): 796-800.

Becker, CM, Sampson, DA, Short, SM, Javaherian, K, Folkman, J & D'Amato, RJ (2006). Short synthetic endostatin peptides inhibit endothelial migration in vitro and endometriosis in a mouse model, *Fertil Steril* 85(1): 71-7.

Bedaiwy, MA, Falcone, T, Sharma, RK, Goldberg, JM, Attaran, M, Nelson, DR & Agarwal, A (2002). Prediction of endometriosis with serum and peritoneal fluid markers: a prospective controlled trial, *Hum Reprod* 17(2): 426-31.

Berkkanoglu, M & Arici, A (2003). Immunology and endometriosis, *Am J Reprod Immunol* 50(1): 48-59.

Braun, DP, Gebel, H, House, R, Rana, N & Dmowski, NP (1996). Spontaneous and induced synthesis of cytokines by peripheral blood monocytes in patients with endometriosis, *Fertil Steril* 65(6): 1125-9.

Brosens, IA (1994). New principles in the management of endometriosis, *Acta Obstet Gynecol Scand Suppl* 159: 18-21.

Chen, QH, Zhou, WD, Su, ZY, Huang, QS, Jiang, JN & Chen, QX Change of proinflammatory cytokines follows certain patterns after induction of endometriosis in a mouse model, *Fertil Steril* 93(5): 1448-54.

Dabrosin, C, Gyorffy, S, Margetts, P, Ross, C & Gauldie, J (2002). Therapeutic effect of angiostatin gene transfer in a murine model of endometriosis, *Am J Pathol* 161(3): 909-18.

Dmowski, WP, Steele, RW & Baker, GF (1981). Deficient cellular immunity in endometriosis, *Am J Obstet Gynecol* 141(4): 377-83.

Dmowski, WP, Gebel, HM & Braun, DP (1994). The role of cell-mediated immunity in pathogenesis of endometriosis, *Acta Obstet Gynecol Scand Suppl* 159: 7-14.

Donnez, J, Smoes, P, Gillerot, S, Casanas-Roux, F & Nisolle, M (1998). Vascular endothelial growth factor (VEGF) in endometriosis, *Hum Reprod* 13(6): 1686-90.

Felson, H, Mc, GJ & Wasserman, P (1960). Stromal endometriosis involving the heart, *Am J Med* 29: 1072-6.

Garcia-Velasco, JA & Arici, A (1999). Interleukin-8 stimulates the adhesion of endometrial stromal cells to fibronectin, *Fertil Steril* 72(2): 336-40.

Giudice, LC (1994). Growth factors and growth modulators in human uterine endometrium: their potential relevance to reproductive medicine, *Fertil Steril* 61(1): 1-17.

Gonzalez-Ramos, R, Van Langendonckt, A, Defrere, S, Lousse, JC, Colette, S, Devoto, L & Donnez, J Involvement of the nuclear factor-kappaB pathway in the pathogenesis of endometriosis, *Fertil Steril* 94(6): 1985-94.

Gonzalez-Ramos, R, Van Langendonckt, A, Defrere, S, Lousse, JC, Colette, S, Devoto, L & Donnez, J (2010). Involvement of the nuclear factor-kappaB pathway in the pathogenesis of endometriosis, *Fertil Steril* 94(6): 1985-94.

Guo, SW, Liu, M, Shen, F & Liu, X Use of mifepristone to treat endometriosis: a review of clinical trials and trial-like studies conducted in China, *Womens Health (Lond Engl)* 7(1): 51-70.

Gupta, S, Agarwal, A, Krajcir, N & Alvarez, JG (2006). Role of oxidative stress in endometriosis, *Reprod Biomed Online* 13(1): 126-34.

Halme, J, Hammond, MG, Hulka, JF, Raj, SG & Talbert, LM (1984). Retrograde menstruation in healthy women and in patients with endometriosis, *Obstet Gynecol* 64(2): 151-4.

Han, S & Sidell, N (2003). RU486-induced growth inhibition of human endometrial cells involves the nuclear factor-kappa B signaling pathway, *J Clin Endocrinol Metab* 88(2): 713-9.

Hill, JA, Faris, HM, Schiff, I & Anderson, DJ (1988). Characterization of leukocyte subpopulations in the peritoneal fluid of women with endometriosis, *Fertil Steril* 50(2): 216-22.

Ho, HN, Wu, MY, Chen, SU, Chao, KH, Chen, CD & Yang, YS (1997). Total antioxidant status and nitric oxide do not increase in peritoneal fluids from women with endometriosis, *Hum Reprod* 12(12): 2810-5.

Hull, ML, Charnock-Jones, DS, Chan, CL, Bruner-Tran, KL, Osteen, KG, Tom, BD, Fan, TP & Smith, SK (2003). Antiangiogenic agents are effective inhibitors of endometriosis, *J Clin Endocrinol Metab* 88(6): 2889-99.

Iwabe, T, Harada, T, Tsudo, T, Tanikawa, M, Onohara, Y & Terakawa, N (1998). Pathogenetic significance of increased levels of interleukin-8 in the peritoneal fluid of patients with endometriosis, *Fertil Steril* 69(5): 924-30.

Jeltsch, M, Kaipainen, A, Joukov, V, Meng, X, Lakso, M, Rauvala, H, Swartz, M, Fukumura, D, Jain, RK & Alitalo, K (1997). Hyperplasia of lymphatic vessels in VEGF-C transgenic mice, *Science* 276(5317): 1423-5.

Jenkins, S, Olive, DL & Haney, AF (1986). Endometriosis: pathogenetic implications of the anatomic distribution, *Obstet Gynecol* 67(3): 335-8.

Joseph, J, Reed, CE & Sahn, SA (1994). Thoracic endometriosis. Recurrence following hysterectomy with bilateral salpingo-oophorectomy and successful treatment with talc pleurodesis, *Chest* 106(6): 1894-6.

Joukov, V, Sorsa, T, Kumar, V, Jeltsch, M, Claesson-Welsh, L, Cao, Y, Saksela, O, Kalkkinen, N & Alitalo, K (1997). Proteolytic processing regulates receptor specificity and activity of VEGF-C, *Embo J* 16(13): 3898-911.

Khorram, O, Taylor, RN, Ryan, IP, Schall, TJ & Landers, DV (1993). Peritoneal fluid concentrations of the cytokine RANTES correlate with the severity of endometriosis, *Am J Obstet Gynecol* 169(6): 1545-9.

Koks, CA, Groothuis, PG, Dunselman, GA, de Goeij, AF & Evers, JL (2000). Adhesion of menstrual endometrium to extracellular matrix: the possible role of integrin alpha(6)beta(1) and laminin interaction, *Mol Hum Reprod* 6(2): 170-7.

Koninckx, PR, Kennedy, SH & Barlow, DH (1998). Endometriotic disease: the role of peritoneal fluid, *Hum Reprod Update* 4(5): 741-51.

Koninckx, PR, Barlow, D & Kennedy, S (1999). Implantation versus infiltration: the Sampson versus the endometriotic disease theory, *Gynecol Obstet Invest* 47 Suppl 1: 3-9; discussion 9-10.

Krikun, G, Hu, Z, Osteen, K, Bruner-Tran, KL, Schatz, F, Taylor, HS, Toti, P, Arcuri, F, Konigsberg, W, Garen, A, Booth, CJ & Lockwood, CJ The immunoconjugate "icon" targets aberrantly expressed endothelial tissue factor causing regression of endometriosis, *Am J Pathol* 176(2): 1050-6.

Kyama, CM, Debrock, S, Mwenda, JM & D'Hooghe, TM (2003). Potential involvement of the immune system in the development of endometriosis, *Reprod Biol Endocrinol* 1: 123.

Kyo, S, Nakamura, M, Kiyono, T, Maida, Y, Kanaya, T, Tanaka, M, Yatabe, N & Inoue, M (2003). Successful immortalization of endometrial glandular cells with normal structural and functional characteristics, *Am J Pathol* 163(6): 2259-69.

Laird, SM, Tuckerman, EM, Saravelos, H & Li, TC (1996). The production of tumour necrosis factor alpha (TNF-alpha) by human endometrial cells in culture, *Hum Reprod* 11(6): 1318-23.

Laird, SM, Tuckerman, EM, Cork, BA & Li, TC (2000). Expression of nuclear factor kappa B in human endometrium; role in the control of interleukin 6 and leukaemia inhibitory factor production, *Mol Hum Reprod* 6(1): 34-40.

Le, JM & Vilcek, J (1989). Interleukin 6: a multifunctional cytokine regulating immune reactions and the acute phase protein response, *Lab Invest* 61(6): 588-602.

Lebovic, DI, Bentzien, F, Chao, VA, Garrett, EN, Meng, YG & Taylor, RN (2000). Induction of an angiogenic phenotype in endometriotic stromal cell cultures by interleukin-1beta, *Mol Hum Reprod* 6(3): 269-75.

Lebovic, DI, Mueller, MD & Taylor, RN (2001). Immunobiology of endometriosis, *Fertil Steril* 75(1): 1-10.

Lessey, BA, Damjanovich, L, Coutifaris, C, Castelbaum, A, Albelda, SM & Buck, CA (1992). Integrin adhesion molecules in the human endometrium. Correlation with the normal and abnormal menstrual cycle, *J Clin Invest* 90(1): 188-95.

Lin, YJ, Lai, MD, Lei, HY & Wing, LY (2006). Neutrophils and macrophages promote angiogenesis in the early stage of endometriosis in a mouse model, *Endocrinology* 147(3): 1278-86.

McLaren, J, Prentice, A, Charnock-Jones, DS, Millican, SA, Muller, KH, Sharkey, AM & Smith, SK (1996). Vascular endothelial growth factor is produced by peritoneal fluid macrophages in endometriosis and is regulated by ovarian steroids, *J Clin Invest* 98(2): 482-9.

McLaren, J, Prentice, A, Charnock-Jones, DS & Smith, SK (1996). Vascular endothelial growth factor (VEGF) concentrations are elevated in peritoneal fluid of women with endometriosis, *Hum Reprod* 11(1): 220-3.

McLaren, J (2000). Vascular endothelial growth factor and endometriotic angiogenesis, *Hum Reprod Update* 6(1): 45-55.

Mettler, L, Volkov, NI, Kulakov, VI, Jurgensen, A & Parwaresch, MR (1996). Lymphocyte subsets in the endometrium of patients with endometriosis throughout the menstrual cycle, *Am J Reprod Immunol* 36(6): 342-8.

Mol, BW, Bayram, N, Lijmer, JG, Wiegerinck, MA, Bongers, MY, van der Veen, F & Bossuyt, PM (1998). The performance of CA-125 measurement in the detection of endometriosis: a meta-analysis, *Fertil Steril* 70(6): 1101-8.

Monckedieck, V, Sannecke, C, Husen, B, Kumbartski, M, Kimmig, R, Totsch, M, Winterhager, E & Grummer, R (2009). Progestins inhibit expression of MMPs and of angiogenic factors in human ectopic endometrial lesions in a mouse model, *Mol Hum Reprod* 15(10): 633-43.

Moretta, A, Sivori, S, Vitale, M, Pende, D, Morelli, L, Augugliaro, R, Bottino, C & Moretta, L (1995). Existence of both inhibitory (p58) and activatory (p50) receptors for HLA-C molecules in human natural killer cells, *J Exp Med* 182(3): 875-84.

Murphy, AA, Palinski, W, Rankin, S, Morales, AJ & Parthasarathy, S (1998). Macrophage scavenger receptor(s) and oxidatively modified proteins in endometriosis, *Fertil Steril* 69(6): 1085-91.

Nalini Santanam, NK, Celia Dominguez, John A. Rock, Sampath Parthasarathy, Ana A. Murphy (2003). Antioxidant supplementation reduces total chemokines and inflammatory cytokines in women with enodmetriosis, *Fertility and Sterility* 80: s32-s33.

Nap, AW, Griffioen, AW, Dunselman, GA, Bouma-Ter Steege, JC, Thijssen, VL, Evers, JL & Groothuis, PG (2004). Antiangiogenesis therapy for endometriosis, *J Clin Endocrinol Metab* 89(3): 1089-95.

Nisolle, M, Casanas-Roux, F, Anaf, V, Mine, JM & Donnez, J (1993). Morphometric study of the stromal vascularization in peritoneal endometriosis, *Fertil Steril* 59(3): 681-4.

Oosterlynck, DJ, Cornillie, FJ, Waer, M, Vandeputte, M & Koninckx, PR (1991). Women with endometriosis show a defect in natural killer activity resulting in a decreased cytotoxicity to autologous endometrium, *Fertil Steril* 56(1): 45-51.

Oosterlynck, DJ, Meuleman, C, Sobis, H, Vandeputte, M & Koninckx, PR (1993). Angiogenic activity of peritoneal fluid from women with endometriosis, *Fertil Steril* 59(4): 778-82.

Oosterlynck, DJ, Meuleman, C, Waer, M & Koninckx, PR (1994). Transforming growth factor-beta activity is increased in peritoneal fluid from women with endometriosis, *Obstet Gynecol* 83(2): 287-92.

Oral, E, Olive, DL & Arici, A (1996). The peritoneal environment in endometriosis, *Hum Reprod Update* 2(5): 385-98.

Ota, H, Igarashi, S & Tanaka, T (2001). Xanthine oxidase in eutopic and ectopic endometrium in endometriosis and adenomyosis, *Fertil Steril* 75(4): 785-90.

Robert, M (1919). Uber den staud der frage der adenomyosites adenomyoma in allemeinen und adenomyonetitis sarcomatosa, *Zentralbl Gynakol* 36: 745-59

Rokitansky, CV (1860). Ueber Uterusdrusen-Neubildung in Uterus- und Ovarial-Sarcomen, *Ztschr kk Gesselsh Aerzte Wien* 16: 577.

Salamonsen, LA & Woolley, DE (1996). Matrix metalloproteinases in normal menstruation, *Hum Reprod* 11 Suppl 2: 124-33.

Sampson, J (1921). Perforating hemorrhagic (chocolate) cysts of the ovary, *Arch Surg* (3): 245-323.

Steele, RW, Dmowski, WP & Marmer, DJ (1984). Immunologic aspects of human endometriosis, *Am J Reprod Immunol* 6(1): 33-6.

Tariverdian, N, Siedentopf, F, Rucke, M, Blois, SM, Klapp, BF, Kentenich, H & Arck, PC (2009). Intraperitoneal immune cell status in infertile women with and without endometriosis, *J Reprod Immunol* 80(1-2): 80-90.

Thibodeau, LL, Prioleau, GR, Manuelidis, EE, Merino, MJ & Heafner, MD (1987). Cerebral endometriosis. Case report, *J Neurosurg* 66(4): 609-10.

Umezawa, M, Sakata, C, Tanaka, N, Kudo, S, Tabata, M, Takeda, K, Ihara, T & Sugamata, M (2008). Cytokine and chemokine expression in a rat endometriosis is similar to that in human endometriosis, *Cytokine* 43(2): 105-9.

van Furth, R, Raeburn, JA & van Zwet, TL (1979). Characteristics of human mononuclear phagocytes, *Blood* 54(2): 485-500.

Van Langendonckt, A, Casanas-Roux, F & Donnez, J (2002). Oxidative stress and peritoneal endometriosis, *Fertil Steril* 77(5): 861-70.

Vigano, P, Gaffuri, B, Somigliana, E, Busacca, M, Di Blasio, AM & Vignali, M (1998). Expression of intercellular adhesion molecule (ICAM)-1 mRNA and protein is enhanced in endometriosis versus endometrial stromal cells in culture, *Mol Hum Reprod* 4(12): 1150-6.

Vlahos, NF, Gregoriou, O, Deliveliotou, A, Perrea, D, Vlachos, A, Zhao, Y, Lai, J & Creatsas, G Effect of pentoxifylline on vascular endothelial growth factor C and flk-1 expression on endometrial implants in the rat endometriosis model, *Fertil Steril* 93(4): 1316-23.

Wang, Y, Sharma, RK, Falcone, T, Goldberg, J & Agarwal, A (1997). Importance of reactive oxygen species in the peritoneal fluid of women with endometriosis or idiopathic infertility, *Fertil Steril* 68(5): 826-30.

Wilson, TJ, Hertzog, PJ, Angus, D, Munnery, L, Wood, EC & Kola, I (1994). Decreased natural killer cell activity in endometriosis patients: relationship to disease pathogenesis, *Fertil Steril* 62(5): 1086-8.

Wu, MY, Yang, JH, Chao, KH, Hwang, JL, Yang, YS & Ho, HN (2000). Increase in the expression of killer cell inhibitory receptors on peritoneal natural killer cells in women with endometriosis, *Fertil Steril* 74(6): 1187-91.

Zeitvogel, A, Baumann, R & Starzinski-Powitz, A (2001). Identification of an invasive, N-cadherin-expressing epithelial cell type in endometriosis using a new cell culture model, *Am J Pathol* 159(5): 1839-52.

Zeller, JM, Henig, I, Radwanska, E & Dmowski, WP (1987). Enhancement of human monocyte and peritoneal macrophage chemiluminescence activities in women with endometriosis, *Am J Reprod Immunol Microbiol* 13(3): 78-82.

Zhang, RJ, Wild, RA & Ojago, JM (1993). Effect of tumor necrosis factor-alpha on adhesion of human endometrial stromal cells to peritoneal mesothelial cells: an in vitro system, *Fertil Steril* 59(6): 1196-201.

13

Sequential Management with Gonadotropin-Releasing Hormone Agonist and Dienogest of Endometriosis-Associated Uterine Myoma and Adenomyosis

Atsushi Imai*, Hiroshi Takagi, Kazutoshi Matsunami and Satoshi Ichigo
Institute of Endocrine-Related Cancer, Matsunami General Hospital,
Japan

1. Introduction

Uterine leiomyoma and adenomyosis represent the most common benign tumors of the female reproductive system (Levy, 2008; Parker, 2007; Sankaran & Manyonda, 2008). These tumors are estrogen dependent, develop during the reproductive period, and are suppressed with menopause. Traditional treatments for myomas and adenomyosis have been various types of surgical techniques. Medical management of these tumors is an approach that has been used recently and is attractive for many gynecologists because of its relative ease and lack of complications (pelvic organ adhesion) compared with surgery. Indications for therapy are similar to those for surgical removal of these tumors and focus on preserving fertility and/or the patient's desire to maintain her uterus. Medications used include androgens, antiprogestogens (mifepristone), raloxifen, and gonadotropin-releasing hormone agonist (GnRHa) (Levy, 2008; Parker, 2007; Sankaran & Manyonda, 2008; Schweppe, 1999). At present, considering efficiency and safety issues, none of the above agents obtained adequate popularity except for GnRHa. However, GnRHa also have disadvantages including bone loss and menopausal symptoms. The effect of GnRHa is transient and reversal of estrogen deprivation occurs soon after discontinuation of the GnRHa and most myoma and adenomyosis returns to their initial size within several months after discontinuation.

Dienogest is a selective progestin that combines the pharmacologic properties of 19-norprogestins and progesterone derivatives, offering potent progestogenic effects without androgenic, mineral corticoid, or glucocorticoid activity (Harada & Taniguchi, 2010; Sasagawa *et al*, 2008; Sitruk-Ware, 2006). Previous trials demonstrated that dienogest provides effective reductions in endometriosis-associated pelvic pain and laparoscopic measures of pathology (Harada *et al*, 2009; Köhler *et al*, 2010; Schindler *et al*, 2006; Strowitzki *et al*, 2010b). Recently, the new progesterone 2 mg daily demonstrated equivalent efficacy to GnRHa (e.g. buserelin acetate and leuprolide acetate) for relieving the pain of endometriosis in two 24-week, randomized studies (Harada *et al*, 2009; Strowitzki *et al*, 2010a; Strowitzki *et al*, 2010b). Because uterine myoma/adenomyosis and endometriosis have many common

---

* Corresponding author: Institute of Endocrine-Related Cancer, Matsunami General Hospital, Kasamatsu, Japan.

features (Huang *et al*, 2010), these successful trials on endometriosis support that the use of dienogest inhibits myoma and adenomyosis growth. While evaluating superiority of dienogest in women with endometriosis, we have found significant shrinkage of myoma nodes coexisted with endometriosis over several months during an administration of dienogest (Ichigo *et al*, 2011). In this paper, we attempted to prevent their regrowth after discontinuation of GnRHa using dienogest. This retrospective study may be the first study that examined the efficacy and safety of dienogest following GnRHa therapy in perimenopausal women until leading to a natural menopause.

2. Materials and methods

2.1 Reproductive chart review

The data were collected from 13 perimenopausal patients sequentially treated with leuprolide acetate (1.88mg monthly, Takeda Pharmaceutical, Japan) for 6 months and dienogest (2mg/day, Mochida Pharmaceutical, Japan) for 6 months against endometriosis in our patient clinic from January 2008 to May 2011. In this retrospective chart review, we included all perimenopausal patients complicated with a myoma node measuring > 4cm or with adenomyosis measuring >10 cm at the age 46-52 years. Measurements of nodes or total uterine volume using MRI were performed at baseline and during treatment at months 6 and 12. For tecknical reasons, leuprolide acetate was supplied in vials and dienogest in tablets.

Size of myoma or overall uterine was measured at three diameters (transverse, vertical and anterior-posterior) with MRI. Half of multiplied three diameters was accepted as size of myomas and uterus. These measurements were repeated 6 and 12 months after starting the therapy.

2.2 Statistics

Pared t-*t*ests were used to analyze in each size change from baseline. Statitstical significance was defined as $P < 0.05$.

Case No.	Age (years)	Myoma type	Total myoma volume (cm³) (% of baseline)		
			Baseline	After GnRHa treatment	After dienogest treatment
1	48	Intramural	108.6	78.6 (72.2)	80.6 (74.0)
2	49	Intramural	72.8	61.9 (85.0)	58.6 (80.5)
3	46	Intramural (multiple)	45.6	33.6 (73.7)	36.9 (80.9)
4	52	Intramural (multiple)	89.3	42.7 (47.8)	50.9 (57.0)
5#	52	Adenomyosis	117.5	56.3 (47.8)	50.3 (42.8)
6	50	Subserosal	88.7	85.6 (96.5)	81.7 (92.1)
7##	52	Subserosal (multiple)	87.2	43.6 (50.0)	45.2 (51.8)
Average	49.9 ± 2.3		87.1 ± 23.5	57.5 ± 19.3* (67.6 ± 19.5)	57.7 ± 17.3* (68.4 ± 18.1)

Table 1. Myoma volume change during sequential treatment with GnRHa and dienogest

The patients were sequentially treated with leuprolide acetate (1.88mg monthly) for 6 months and dienogest (2mg daily) for 6months. Measurements of nodes using MRI were performed at baseline, during treatment at months 6 (after GnRHa therapy) and 12 (after dienogest therapy).

MRI changes of case 5 are presented as a representative prolile in Fig.1.

Case 7 was submitted to laparotomy at month 8 because of bilateral ovarian abscess. See Fig. 2.

* $P < 0.01$ versus baseline.

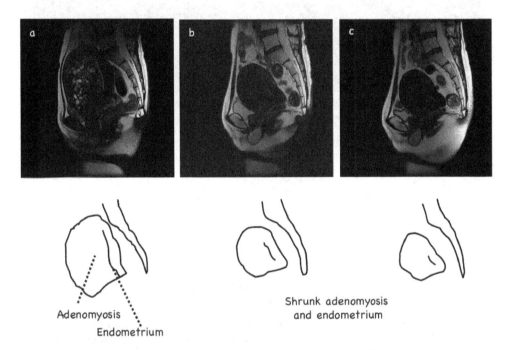

Fig. 1. Total uterine volume change in the patient with myoma during sequential treatment with GnRHa and dienogest (case 6 of Table 1).

The patient was sequentially treated with leuprolide acetate (1.88mg monthly) for 6 months and dienogest (2mg daily) for 6months. Sagittal T2-weighed MR imagings before (a), months 6 (after GnRHa therapy) (b) and 12 (after dienogest therapy)(c)

3. Results

Of 13 endometriosis patients sequentially treated with GnRHa and dienogest, 7 were associated with coexistent myoma node and adenomyosis; 4 intramural and 2 subserosal types and 1 of adenomyosis. Mean age was 49.9 ± 2.3 (46-52)(Table 1). Volume changes of total myoma and adenomyosis are presented as the percentage change from baseline in Table 1. A remarkable reduction in myoma /adenomyosis volume from baseline was noted:

the total volume of myoma/adenomyosis declined to 67.6 ± 19.5 % after GnRHa treatment table 1). During the dienogest-period, myoma volume remained as they shrunk; no regrowth occurred. Fig. 1 showed as a representative profile (case 6 of Table 1). One patient (case 7) discontinued therapy because of an unexpected event, onset on ovarian abscess developed in the endometrioma (see Fig.2).

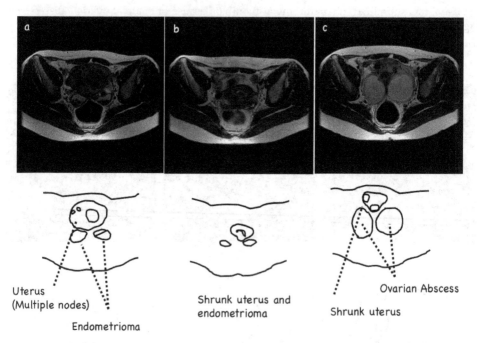

Fig. 2. Bilateral *de novo* ovarian abscesses in a 52-year-old woman with multilobular uterine myoma and bilateral ovarian endometriomas (case 7, table 1).

The patient was treated with leuprolide acetate (1.88mg monthly, Takeda Pharmaceutical, Japan) for 6 months. Axial T2-weighed MR imagings before (a) and after (b) GnRHa treatment showed remarkable shrinkage of uterine myoma and bilateral endometriomas. An attempt to prevent the recurrence submitted the patient to dienogest therapy (2mg daily, Mochida Pharmaceutical, Japan). After two months, she complaint a one-week history of increasing abdominal girth and a two-day history of fever. Axial T2-weighed MR imaging (c) showed two enlarged cystic lesions, one in the left adnexa and the other in the right adnexa. Both lesions were superimposed on the endometrioma with inhomogenous content and the thick wall, while shrunk uterine myoma was detected. There was no history of gynecological interventions including endometrioma aspiration, no had she ever used an intra-uterine device. The clinical and imaging findings and unresponsive to antibiotic therapy proposed the ovarian abscess developed in the endometriomas. At laparotomy, both ovarian cysts were markedly distended and filled with yellow-brown pus, and both ovaries were destroyed by multiple abscess pockets. Histology of the abscess wall confirmed endometriotic nature of the cyst.

4. Discussion

Uterine myoma/adenomyosis and endometriosis have many common features. Both are estrogen-dependent conditions that can often be the source of pelvic pain and menstrual abnormalities. In addition, both have range of symptom severity that is often poorly correlated to preoperative or operative findings, making surgical planning a challenge (Huang et al, 2010). Recently we found significant shrinkage of myoma nodes coexisted with endometriosis over several months during an administration of dienogest (Ichigo et al, 2011). To our knowledge this retrospective study may be the first study that examined the efficacy and safety of sequential management with dienogest following GnRHa therapy in perimenopausal women until leading to a natural menopause.

Many studies have reported the potential usefulness of the hypoestrogenic state induced by GnRHa for treatment of uterine myoma (Levy, 2008; Parker, 2007; Sankaran & Manyonda, 2008). A GnRHa down-regulates the pituitary-ovarian-gonadal axis, leading to suppression of ovarian steroidogenesis. In the present study our patients revealed an average reduction of 57.5 % in myoma volume in response to leuprolide acetae (1.8mg/month). The results are in agreement with those of previous studies (Levy, 2008; Parker, 2007; Parsanezhad *et al*, 2010; Sankaran & Manyonda, 2008). The GnRHa treatment is often associated with so-called ovarian defect symptoms, including vasomotor instability, vaginal dryness, and significant bone loss, which preclude the long-term use of this compound (Levy, 2008; Parker, 2007; Sankaran & Manyonda, 2008). These limit the standard use of GnRHa to 6 months. The regression of uterine or endometriosis volume is not permanent, with returning to their original size or even enlarging more rapidly upon cessation of GnRHa administration. GnRHa, therefore, can only be used in the short term, as temporizing measures in the perimenopausal woman, or pre-operatively to reduce myoma size, influence the type of surgery, restore hemoglobin levels and apparently reduce blood loss at operation (Sankaran & Manyonda, 2008).

There may be profound differences among the available progestins according to their structure, metabolites and pharmacodynamic actions (Harada & Taniguchi, 2010; Sasagawa *et al*, 2008; Sitruk-Ware, 2006). It is therefore inappropriate to consider the various effects of the older and newer progestins as class effects. While it has long been established that estrogen promotes myoma growth, many biochemical and clinical studies suggested that older progestins, without an estrogen component, may be effective in the treatment of endometriosis, but not adenomyosis or myomas (Levy, 2008; Parker, 2007; Sankaran & Manyonda, 2008). The newer progestin dienogest demonstrates a modest suppression of estradiol, representing a potential advantage over other therapies, such as GnRHa, which require estrogen add-back if used longer than 6 months (Harada & Taniguchi, 2010; Strowitzki *et al*, 2010a). Also in contrast to GnRHa, dienogest is not associated with an increased incidence of hot flashes (Strowitzki *et al*, 2010a; Strowitzki *et al*, 2010b). More recently the efficacy and safety of long-term usage of dienogest have been demonstrated in previous controlled studies in a large number of patients with endometriosis (Endrikat *et al*, 2007; Momoeda *et al*, 2009; Schindler *et al*, 2010; Sitruk-Ware, 2006). Our previous paper demonstrated that the use of dienogest have several advantages over GnRHa therapy to manage uterine myoma (Ichigo *et al*, 2011). Management of uterine myoma using dienogest is useful in women for whom temporary reduction in myoma volume is aimed and no surgical intervention is planned for any reason. Women with uterine myoma who have pain, pressure effect, hypermenorrhea, or other types of abnormal uterine bleeding who wish to retain the option of childbirth; women who wish to save their uterus; women who are not fit for surgical intervention; and young women with infertility can take advantage of this type of treatment. However, the total decline in myoma volume and controlling symptoms are greater in GnRHa protocol (Ichigo *et al*, 2011). The benefit of dienogest in controlling symptoms may persist after therapy of GnRHa in perimenopausal women.

In the previous study (Imai *et al*, 2003), because rapid regrowth frequently occurs after the therapy is stopped. we attempted to determine whether GnRHa therapy could lead perimenopausal women carrying symptomatic myomas to the natural onset of the menopause. A retrospective analysis of 145 patients who received GnRHa for 24 weeks demonstrated that after cessation of therapy no menstruation occurred over 25 weeks in women aged over 45 years, with elevated levels of follicle-stimulating hormone (FSH) and luteinising hormone (LH). To extend this observation, we studied prospectively 21 women, aged 45 years and older who had regular menstruation with symptoms attributed to myomas and elevated days 3 - 5 FSH and days 3 - 5 LH levels (> 25 mIU/ml). After discontinuation of GnRHa (leuprorelin acetate, 1.88 mg) therapy for 6 months, menstruation occurred in only two of 21 individuals but the remaining 19 cases had no menstrual bleeding. It is suggested that the rise in early follicular phase serum gonadotrophins, in particular FSH (> 25 mIU/ml), may precede the natural menopause following (or during) GnRHa therapy in older women. Measuring days 3 to 5 serum FSH concentrations may make it easier to decide on the optimal duration of therapy for symptomatic uterine fibroids in perimenopausal women aged > 45 years. However, in other words, approximately 10 % of women failed to become natural menopause.

Regarding an unexpected event of case 7 of table 1, she has no known previous history of pelvic inflammatory disease, IUD, or any surgical intervention, so she was very unlikely to present with ovarian abscess. It shows that an isolated ovarian abscess can develop in an endometrioma without any recognized risk factor. There are different theories about developing an abscess in the endometrioma (Hameed *et al*, 2010; Kavoussi *et al*, 2006). It may be due to an altered immune environment within endometrial glands and stroma. Recent studies have shown that progesterone-like substances enhance the sexual transmission of various pathogens, including bacteria (Huber & Gruber, 2001; Vassiliadou *et al*, 1999). Collection of altered menstrual type of blood in a cystic space in the ovary and can be a suitable culture medium for pathogens. Cystic wall of endometrioma is theoretically weak as compared to normal ovarian epithelium, so it is susceptible to bacterial invasion.

Lastly, we reported successful management of a series of patients with uterine myoma associated with endometriosis by sequential therapy with GnRHa and a progestine dienogest, although based on the finding in patients associated with endometriosis. The follow-up period of our study was too short to consider the recurrence rate of myomas after discontinuation of treatment in all subjects. Although prospective controlled study should be addressed, the use of dienogest treatment following GnRHa discontinuation for perimenopausal women with symptomatic uterine myoma or adenomyosis should be considered before choosing a more invasive interventions.

5. Conclusion

High recurrence rate rapidly after finishing GnRHa leads us to examine the efficacy of sequential management with GnRHa and dienogest in perimenopausal women with endometrisosis-associated uterine myoma. Consideration of GnRHa advantages on myoma shrinkage and low incidence of dienogest-induced adverse events may lead to long-term management of perimenopausal women with myoma and adenomyosis.

6. Conflict of interest

The authors declare that they have no conflict of interest.

7. References

Endrikat, J.; Graeser, T., Mellinger, U., Ertan, K. & Holz, C. (2007) A multicenter, prospective, randomized, double-blind, placebo-controlled study to investigate the efficacy of a continuous-combined hormone therapy preparation containing 1mg estradiol valerate/2mg dienogest on hot flushes in postmenopausal women. *Maturitas* Vol.58, pp. 201-201, ISSN 0378-5122

Hameed, A.; Mehta, V. & Sinha, P. (2010) A rare case of de novo gigantic ovarian abscess within an endometrioma. *Yale Journal of Biology and Medicine* Vol.83, pp. 73-75, ISSN 0044-0086

Harada, T.; Momoeda, M., Taketani, Y., Aso, T., Fukunaga, M., Hagino, H. & Terakawa, N. (2009) Dienogest is as effective as intranasal buserelin acetate for the relief of pain symptoms associated with endometriosis--a randomized, double-blind, multicenter, controlled trial. *Fertility and Sterility* Vol.91, pp. 675-681, ISSN 0015-0282

Harada, T. & Taniguchi, F. (2010) Dienogest: a new therapeutic agent for the treatment of endometriosis. *Women's Health* Vol.6, pp. 27-35, ISSN 1745-5057

Huang, J.; Lathi, R., Lemyre, M., Rodriguez, H., Nezhat, C. & Nezhat, C. (2010) Coexistence of endometriosis in women with symptomatic leiomyomas. *Fertility and Sterility* Vol.94, pp. 720-723, ISSN 0015-0282

Huber, J. & Gruber, C. (2001) Immunological and dermatological impact of progesterone. *Gynecological Endocrinology* Vol.15 (Suppl 6), pp. 18-212, ISSN 0951-3590

Ichigo, S.; Takagi, H., Matsunami, K., Suzuki, N. & Imai, A. (2011) Beneficial effects of dienogest on uterine myoma volume: a retrospective controlled study comparing with gonadotropin-releasing hormone agonist. *Archives of Gynecology and Obstetrics* Vol.Epub ahead of print, ISSN 0932-0067

Imai, A.; Sugiyama, M., Furui, T. & Tamaya, T. (2003) Treatment of perimenopausal women with uterine myoma: successful use of a depot GnRH agonist leading to a natural menopause. Journal of Obstetrics and Gynaecology Vol.23, pp 518-520, ISSN 0144-3615

Kavoussi, S.; Pearlman, M., Burke, W. & Lebovic, D. (2006) Endometrioma complicated by tubo-ovarian abscess in a woman with bacterial vaginosis. *Infectious Disease in Obstetrics and Gynecology* Vol.2006, pp. 1-3,

Köhler, G.; Faustmann, T., Gerlinger, C., Seitz, C. & Mueck, A. (2010) A dose-ranging study to determine the efficacy and safety of 1, 2, and 4mg of dienogest daily for endometriosis. *International Journal of Gynaecology and Obstetrics* Vol.108, pp. 21-25, ISSN: 0020-7292

Levy, B. (2008) Modern management of uterine fibroids. *Acta Obstetricia et Gynecologica Scandinavica* Vol.87, pp. 812-823, ISSN 1600-0412

Momoeda, M.; Harada, T., Terakawa, N., Aso, T., Fukunaga, M., Hagino, H. & Taketani, Y. (2009) Long-term use of dienogest for the treatment of endometriosis. *Journal of Obstetric and Gynaecological Research* Vol.35, pp. 1069-1076, ISSN 13418076

Parker, W. (2007) Uterine myomas: management. *Fertility and Sterility* Vol.88, pp. 255-271, ISSN 0015-0282

Parsanezhad, M.; Azmoon, M., Alborzi, S., Rajaeefard, A., Zarei, A., Kazerooni, T., Frank, V. & Schmidt, E. (2010) A randomized, controlled clinical trial comparing the effects of aromatase inhibitor (letrozole) and gonadotropin-releasing hormone agonist (triptorelin) on uterine leiomyoma volume and hormonal status. *Fertility and Sterility* Vol.93, pp. 192-198, ISSN 0015-0282

Sankaran, S. & Manyonda, I. (2008) Medical management of fibroids. *Best Practice & Research Clinical Obstetrics & Gynaecology* Vol.22, pp. 655-676, ISSN 1521-6934

Sasagawa, S.; Shimizu, Y., Kami, H., Takeuchi, T., Mita, S., Imada, K., Kato, S. & Mizuguchi, K. (2008) Dienogest is a selective progesterone receptor agonist in transactivation analysis with potent oral endometrial activity due to its efficient pharmacokinetic profile. *Steroids* Vol.73, pp. 222-231, ISSN 0039-128X

Schindler, A.; Christensen, B., Henkel, A., Oettel, M. & Moore, C. (2006) High-dose pilot study with the novel progestogen dienogestin patients with endometriosis. *Gynecolical Endocrinology* Vol.22, pp. 9-17, ISSN 0951-3590

Schindler, A.; Henkel, A., Moore, C. & Oettel, M. (2010) Effect and safety of high-dose dienogest (20 mg/day) in the treatment of women with endometriosis. *Archives of Gynecology and Obstetrics* Vol.282, pp. 507-514, ISSN 0932-0067

Schweppe, K. (1999) Progestins and uterine leiomyoma. *Gynecologycal Endocrinology* Vol.13 Suppl 4, pp. 21-24, ISSN 0951-3590

Sitruk-Ware, R. (2006) New progestagens for contraceptive use. *Human Reproduction Update* Vol.12, pp. 169-178, ISSN 1355-4786

Strowitzki, T.; Faustmann, T., Gerlinger, C. & Seitz, C. (2010a) Dienogest in the treatment of endometriosis-associated pelvic pain: a 12-week, randomized, double-blind, placebo-controlled study. *European Journal of Obstetrics & Gynecology and Reproductive Biology* Vol.151, pp. 193-198, ISSN 0301-2115

Strowitzki, T.; Marr, J., Gerlinger, C., Faustmann, T. & Seitz, C. (2010b) Dienogest is as effective as leuprolide acetate in treating the painful symptoms of endometriosis: a 24-week, randomized, multicentre, open-label trial. *Human Reproduction Update* Vol.25, pp. 633-641, ISSN 1355-4786

Vassiliadou, N.; Tucker, L. & Anderson, D. (1999) Progesterone-induced inhibition of chemokine receptor expression on peripheral blood mononuclear cells correlates with reduced HIV-1 infectability in vitro. *Journal of Immunology* Vol.162, pp. 7510-7518, ISSN 0022-1767

Permissions

The contributors of this book come from diverse backgrounds, making this book a truly international effort. This book will bring forth new frontiers with its revolutionizing research information and detailed analysis of the nascent developments around the world.

We would like to thank Koel Chaudhury and Baidyanath Chakravarty, for lending their expertise to make the book truly unique. They have played a crucial role in the development of this book. Without their invaluable contribution this book wouldn't have been possible. They have made vital efforts to compile up to date information on the varied aspects of this subject to make this book a valuable addition to the collection of many professionals and students.

This book was conceptualized with the vision of imparting up-to-date information and advanced data in this field. To ensure the same, a matchless editorial board was set up. Every individual on the board went through rigorous rounds of assessment to prove their worth. After which they invested a large part of their time researching and compiling the most relevant data for our readers. Conferences and sessions were held from time to time between the editorial board and the contributing authors to present the data in the most comprehensible form. The editorial team has worked tirelessly to provide valuable and valid information to help people across the globe.

Every chapter published in this book has been scrutinized by our experts. Their significance has been extensively debated. The topics covered herein carry significant findings which will fuel the growth of the discipline. They may even be implemented as practical applications or may be referred to as a beginning point for another development. Chapters in this book were first published by InTech; hereby published with permission under the Creative Commons Attribution License or equivalent.

The editorial board has been involved in producing this book since its inception. They have spent rigorous hours researching and exploring the diverse topics which have resulted in the successful publishing of this book. They have passed on their knowledge of decades through this book. To expedite this challenging task, the publisher supported the team at every step. A small team of assistant editors was also appointed to further simplify the editing procedure and attain best results for the readers.

Our editorial team has been hand-picked from every corner of the world. Their multi-ethnicity adds dynamic inputs to the discussions which result in innovative outcomes. These outcomes are then further discussed with the researchers and contributors who give their valuable feedback and opinion regarding the same. The feedback is then collaborated with the researches and they are edited in a comprehensive manner to aid the understanding of the subject.

Apart from the editorial board, the designing team has also invested a significant amount of their time in understanding the subject and creating the most relevant covers. They scrutinized every image to scout for the most suitable representation of the subject and create an appropriate cover for the book.

The publishing team has been involved in this book since its early stages. They were actively engaged in every process, be it collecting the data, connecting with the contributors or procuring relevant information. The team has been an ardent support to the editorial, designing and production team. Their endless efforts to recruit the best for this project, has resulted in the accomplishment of this book. They are a veteran in the field of academics and their pool of knowledge is as vast as their experience in printing. Their expertise and guidance has proved useful at every step. Their uncompromising quality standards have made this book an exceptional effort. Their encouragement from time to time has been an inspiration for everyone.

The publisher and the editorial board hope that this book will prove to be a valuable piece of knowledge for researchers, students, practitioners and scholars across the globe.

List of Contributors

Victor Chaban
Charles R. Drew University of Medicine and Science and University of California, Los Angeles, USA

Hendi Hendarto
Dept. of Obstetrics & Gynecology Faculty of Medicine, University of Airlangga / Dr. Soetomo Hospital, Surabaya, Indonesia

Yoriko Yamashita and Shinya Toyokuni
Nagoya University Graduate School of Medicine, Japan

Saikat K. Jana, Priyanka Banerjee, Shyam Thangaraju, Baidyanath Chakravarty and Koel Chaudhury
Indian Institute of Technology, Kharagpur, India

Aixingzi Aili, Ding Yan, Hu Wenjing, Yang Xinhua and Hanikezi Tuerxun
Xinjiang Medical University, China

Ionara Barcelos
University of West Parana, Da Vinci - Reproductive Medicine, Brazil

Paula Navarro
University of Sao Paulo, University of Sao Paulo - Ribeirao Preto, Brazil

Veljko Vlaisavljević, Marko Došen and Borut Kovačič
Department of Reproductive Medicine and Gynecologic Endocrinology, Clinics for Gynecology and Perinatology, University Clinical Center Maribor, Slovenia

Michele Cioffi and Maria Teresa Vietri
Department of General Pathology, Faculty of Medicine and Surgery of Second University of Naples, Naples, Italy

Rosario Francesco Grasso, Riccardo Del Vescovo, Roberto Luigi Cazzato and Bruno Beomonte Zobel
Department of Radiology, Campus Bio-Medico University of Rome, Italy

Shalini Jain Bagaria
Department of Obstetrics & Gynecology, UCMS & GTB Hospital, Dilshad Garden, Delhi, India

Darshana D. Rasalkar and Bhawan K. Paunipagar
Department of Imaging and Interventional Radiology, The Chinese University of Hong Kong, Prince of Wales Hospital, Hong Kong

Elham Pourmatroud
Ahvaz Jundishapur University of Medical Science (AJUMS), Iran

Tao Zhang, Gene Chi Wai Man and Chi Chiu Wang
Department of Obstetrics and Gynaecology, The Chinese University of Hong Kong, Prince of Wales Hospital, Shatin, New Territories, Hong Kong

Atsushi Imai, Hiroshi Takagi, Kazutoshi Matsunami and Satoshi Ichigo
Institute of Endocrine-Related Cancer, Matsunami General Hospital, Japan